Bonnie!

All the

[signature] Rob Hawke

Kicking
Cancer's
Ass

A Light-Hearted Guide
to the Fight of Your Life

ROBERT HAWKE

ISBN 978-0-9876924-0-5

Dedication

**To all those who have the courage to get through this,
but don't know it yet.**

Table of Contents

Acknowledgments

Act 1: Getting Ready

Chapter 1 — You're Going to Get through This 1

Chapter 2 — Getting the News 11

Chapter 3 — Battening Down the Hatches 23

Act 2: Going Through It

Chapter 4 — Getting Yourself Educated 34

Chapter 5 — Testing... Testing... 47

Chapter 6 — Prepping for Surgery or Treatment 64

Chapter 7 — My Hospital Experience 74

Act 3: Recovering

Chapter 8 — Recovery: When you First Get Home 82

Chapter 9 — Recovery: Further Down the Road 89

Chapter 10 — A Work In Progress 104

Chapter 11 — Rebuilding Your Life 111

Chapter 12 — Strategies for the Future 120

Chapter 13 — But I Thought I Was Done! 129

Act 4: For Caregivers

Chapter 14 — Before Treatment 132

Chapter 15 — At the Hospital 140

Chapter 16 — At Home 155

About the Author 163

Acknowledgments

There are so many generous people who have contributed to this book and my journey back to a healthy life. I would like to thank my remarkable Mom and Dad, my brothers Mark and Dave, the mighty Gord Oxley, Jane Luk, Louis Vitela, my awesome nephews, Sandi Sloan, Dr Kenneth Florence, Dr. Kate Hays, Dr. Jeremy Freeman, Dr. Kim McKenzie, Dr. Paul Walfish, Dr Andrew Matthew, Michael Cohen, Nadine Cross, Gail Mitchell, Dr. Dante Morra, Ron Proulx, everyone at the Centre For Innovation in Complex Care, all of the stakeholders and team members of The Patient Empowerment Program, The Bad Dog Theatre Company, and Mount Sinai Hospital in Toronto.

Special thanks to my wonderful wife Cindy Fajardo, for gently encouraging me every step of the way.

Chapter 1

You're Going to Get through This

In this chapter:

Hi, my name is Rob
You're going to get through this
The two big questions
We're in this together

Hi,

I'm sorry you have to read this book. I know that it might seem a bit crazy for an author to say that, but I am sorry. You may have just received a diagnosis of cancer that came as a real shock or perhaps you're a bit further down the road. Either way, my heart goes out to you in hopes that you will be healthy and happy again.

It wasn't so long ago that I went on this journey they call "having cancer" as well. It took me completely by surprise and was not a pleasant experience but I am better now. And although I'm missing a gland that I didn't even know existed, I am OK. In fact, I'm better than OK, I'm happy and well, and I certainly wish these things for you.

I hope that in this book, you will find some things that

will make this path easier for you. When I was diagnosed, and in the days that followed, I was amazed at how little I knew about my own condition and how ill-prepared I was. I blundered through the experience the best I could but I really could have used some kind of guidebook that would help me through the experience. I remember being in my humble apartment a few days after surgery and thinking to myself "Someone has to tell people what this is like!" At that point, I realized that I was going to do my best to help folks going through this experience.

I hope this book lets you know that you are not alone. You might find yourself feeling isolated and be convinced that "no one can possibly know what this is like" or that you are "having a truly unique experience that no one can relate to." I felt much the same way. However, there are literally thousands of us who are putting on a stiff upper lip and going on with the day while trying like hell to ignore that fact that we are staring down a diagnosis of the big "C". With all of us going through such a common experience, it's clear then that even though we may feel alone, we are connected with a great tide of humanity that is having a similar experience.

Just to let you know, I have a background in comedy; not surprisingly, one of my favourite coping mechanisms is humour. Throughout this book, I'll use humour sporadically to get a point across or just to lighten things up a bit. I'm not doing this out of disrespect, in fact quite the opposite: I respect what you're going through so much that I think you should use every tool you have to get through this, and that includes humour.

The medical odds are that you will survive this experience.

When I was first diagnosed, I felt like there were so many

things I didn't know, so many things I was scared of and so much in my life that was out of my control. I felt completely overwhelmed, but in time, I managed to get through my diagnosis, treatment and recovery. Obviously, I don't know what the future holds for you, but I do know that we live in a time when there are more resources available for people like us than ever before. Once you are out the other side, you will still crave chocolate, you will still be yourself, you will still love and be loved.

This is one of life's journeys, and a big one at that. This is not to be taken lightly like a trip to the corner store; it is, in fact, an epic trip that involves a great deal of change, and will require courage, faith, love and strength. Along the way you will probably experience laughter, tears, frustration, pain, relief and every other emotion that Meryl Streep goes through in a movie.

I am not pretending to have all the answers to your situation in this book. I am the first to admit that there are many things I don't know; for instance, I am not a doctor and I don't have any letters after my name, but I have lived through cancer at a young age (I keep telling myself 40 is still young. Please don't tell me otherwise.) and shortly after that I was the primary caregiver for someone who was diagnosed with the disease. Many times I wished I had someone with me to tell me what was going on, to help me out and offer me advice when something came up, or just somebody who had gone through it who could give me a few pointers along the way. It is my hope that this book does that for you and that maybe in some small way, it makes your difficult trip easier.

"Cancer is a word, not a sentence."
—John Diamond

Let's Start at the End...

I was going to begin at the beginning, but you are living that right now, so for a second I'd like to jump to the end of the story, so you know how it finishes.

Imagine if you will a time in the future when you have your health back, when you feel good again, when you have adjusted to the changes in your life and have your feet planted firmly on the ground. A time after you have wrestled with experiences that most folks wouldn't even begin to know how to deal with and you have emerged victorious. Now imagine that all the resources you need, all the love, support, education and terrific medical care will come your way. You may not be there yet, but you will be.

Many thousands of us survive cancer every single year. Often, we are stronger than we were, have more depth, more love, more appreciation, and more soul to our lives than we did before.

You might think I'm coming at this with blind optimism, saying, "Hey it's all going to be great! Cancer is a walk in the park!" I'm not implying that at all. What I am saying is that each day of this journey, you will go a little further along the road to healing. I know that it seems trite to put it that way, but you will get through this. The old adage of a journey of a thousand miles beginning with a single step is certainly true here, and although you might feel pissed off, sad, hurt, or all of the above, it is right on schedule for what is expected of you right now.

There are many different forms of cancer and many varying degrees of sickness and health that go with it. With all these disparities in our collective experience, how can we help each other through this? Well, even though your body may be different than mine and our levels of health may be different, I also know that we are

4

linked by this; we all go through similar experiences emotionally, socially and sometimes spiritually. It is in those experiences that we can share commonalities and learn from each other to make the road easier as we go.

"The only courage that matters is the kind that gets you from one moment to the next."
—**Mignon McLaughlin**

Cancer survival rates in virtually every country in the world are going up. At the same time the incidence rate of many kinds of cancer are going down. The stats are that roughly a third of the people in the industrialized world will deal with a diagnosis at some point in their lives. A third. That's huge. Is this a reason to be hopeful? Sure. If a full third of the population will get this, there must be thousands upon thousands of examples of people living through this and getting on with their lives.

Medical treatments are getting better all the time. This disease was once considered a death sentence, and the word itself was barely whispered in public. These days, our ability to deal with cancer as a condition that we can treat effectively and proactively becomes stronger every day.

Where Will I Get the Resources?

Becoming healthy again will require that you use a lot of your internal resources. Your "muscles" of courage, determination and hope will certainly get a workout and of course you will also get help from family and friends as well. There are many around you right now who will be able to offer advice on a good doctor to see, an informative book to read or even a shoulder to cry on when things are tough. The point is, you probably have more resources right now than you think you have, and on the occasion when you feel like you are all used up, something just might magically appear to help you out. So, since the odds are that you are going to get through this and we know that there are many resources at your disposal, let's get started...

The Two Big Questions

The two questions that really demanded an answer for me during this time were "Is this my fault" and "Why the hell did this happen to me?" Of all the questions that rolled through my head while I was pretending to work or trying to sleep, these two were the toughest for me to deal with. Let's have a look at them now...

Question #1: Is this my fault?

There has been a great deal of discussion about the nature of reality itself and whether or not we create the circumstances of our lives through our thoughts and feelings. This belief in our responsibility for virtually everything that happens to us has grown ever more prevalent in the last couple of decades.

Some would have us believe that *everything* we experience is a result of our thought processes. Because I believed this to a degree and I had consciously manifested some circumstances in my life before, I felt really guilty after I got my diagnosis. My thought process went like this: "If I create everything in my life through my thoughts and feelings, then certainly, every aspect of my health is my responsibility also. And thus I clearly have given myself cancer in some way."

So, not only did I have to deal with the diagnosis of a

disease but I also felt remarkably guilty just for having it! Gosh, I must have been a really bad person to have created cancer for myself. Frankly, I don't know if there is any validity to the belief that we create every aspect of our own reality or not, but there is hard medical research about what causes this disease, and *that* we *can* talk about.

So what do we know about what actually causes cancer? The three major contributing factors are…
1: Your genetic background.
2: Your environment.
3: Your lifestyle.

You might notice that you have very little control over both your genetic background and to some degree, the environment you live in. Getting mad at yourself for any genetic tendency you might have to get a disease makes about as much sense as getting mad at yourself for the colour of your eyes or the fact that you might not be as tall as you'd like. We can't help what we have in our genetic code. At this point in human experience it's impossible for us to alter the DNA in every cell we have in order to not get a certain disease. We clearly aren't responsible for the specific genetic pool in which we were born.

Now let's talk about the environment. We need to remind ourselves that our world has become more chemically complex and polluted with each generation for hundreds of years now. In an urban environment, there are many chemicals in the air, water, and in the ground that we can do nothing about. In fact, artificial materials are so prevalent that we get excited when something is 100% natural! We live in a world where we are bombarded with radiation, radio waves, electrical currents and old Uncle Jim's off-colour jokes. So, it's not surprising if we have health issues when the vast majority of us live in an environment that at best could be called "less than ideal." Why do I bring all this up? Because...

It's not your fault.

I am all for us taking responsibility for our lives but there are some things we just don't control. Yes, there are lifestyle choices that have a profound affect on whether or not we are healthy or sick. Things like quitting smoking, having a healthy diet full of greens, and getting exercise all reduce the chances that we will have major health issues in our lives, but some of the causes are just beyond are control. So, if you're feeling guilty or responsible, let yourself off the hook. It's alright. As Robin Williams said to Matt Damon in *Good Will Hunting*, "It's not your fault."

Question #2: Why the hell did this happen to me?

I don't know. I have no idea why this disease came into your life and I have no idea why it came into mine. I have thought about this for a long time and not only can I not give you a definitive answer, it is unlikely that anyone else can either. Sure, people may talk about likelihoods and percentages, but a definite cause may prove illusive. This drove me a bit crazy for a while because I really wanted to look at some aspect of my life and say 'Hey, this is the thing that caused my cancer!" but I did not have that experience at all. In fact, not one of my medical professionals even attempted to tell me what had caused my sickness. I really wanted to know what I'd eaten, smelled, or bathed in that had given me the disease. Some of the things I had wondered about were too much TV, too much cereal and even fabric made in China. If any of these things caused cancer, then a *lot* of the folks I hung out with would have had the disease. I drove myself crazy with this for a while until I finally just accepted that I might never know why.

In this situation, it's common for us to want to lay blame, point a finger or kick the crap out of whatever did this to us. More often than not we are left with vague conjecture, like "Hey it runs in your family and you use plastic wrap," which does not offer much in the way of closure, to say the least.

So who do we blame? I was really angry at myself for a long time, thinking I had done something wrong. Folks even told me that maybe I got cancer because I am naturally enthusiastic and emotionally intense (which is, of course, ridiculous). Many times we have to come to terms with the fact that we will never truly know why and how we came to deal with this. It can be like wondering why a tornado randomly smashed your house to bits but left your neighbor's place pristine and beautiful, with the happy dog still tied to the picket fence. At these times of loss, we look to different explanations for comfort and solace: "It was God's will", "It's all part of a plan", "This is just random stuff that happens on occasion", or even 'I am paying back Karma for stealing a chocolate bar when I was eight.'

I don't know which of these answers, if any, is correct, but I do know that we as humans feel there has to be a reason for things. However intelligent we are, though, occasionally there are some things we just don't know. And not knowing makes us want to reach up to the sky and yell "Tell me what I did! Tell me who to blame! Tell me what I did to deserve this!" We wait for a response...and sometimes, there is no answer, which can be the cruelest answer of all. In fact, occasionally I still wrestle with this myself at 3 AM. There are many of us who have asked the same thing in the dark of night. You are not alone in your alone-ness. Thousands of us are together in this, doing our best to muddle through each step of the way. Those of us who have already gone through the experience once asked the same questions you are and now we're rebuilding our lives. We wish the same thing for you. So let's get to it.

Chapter 2

Getting the News

In this chapter:

A shock to the system
Get ready to notice the "Big C"
Let it out!
The Fight or Flight response
Three strategies for the early days
How to tell people

Getting the News

You may have received word of your condition face to face in your doctor's office or you may have gotten the news over the phone. Either way, I'm guessing it came as a surprise. Very few people expect to be told they have cancer and it can come as a real shock to your system. People often talk about how when they hear news that is really impactful, that the world kind of spins or looks a bit different. This was how it was for me. I wasn't told outright that I had the disease but all of a sudden the percentage chance of me having a malignancy went from forty to eighty percent. I walked out of the doctor's office onto College St., managed to buy a coffee, and sat there stunned for a while. I mean cancer? Come on! What are the odds of that? I knew at that moment that the world was going to be different for me.

After I sat stupefied for a while, the news sunk in a bit and I got myself home. As the days went by, something kind of strange happened: I noticed that the word cancer was virtually everywhere. It got kind of ridiculous for a while. Allow me to illustrate this with a sketch:

You're sitting on your couch on a relaxing Tuesday evening, watching a rather dramatic ballgame on TV. It's gone into extra innings, the crowd is hushed and you are completely mesmerized by the action.

TV Commentator #1
Well now Fernandez is coming to bat. He steps into the batters box and the first pitch goes by. It's a strike!

TV Commentator #2:
You know Bob, Fernandez hasn't been doing so well this year. His Batting Average is down from .303 to .186!

TV Commentator #1:
Here's another pitch. It's a swing and a miss. Oh and he's struck out!

TV Commentator #2:
He sure did Bob. These Milwaukee pitchers are giving him so much trouble they're almost like a *cancer* to him.

You grimace and change the channel. Over to Fox News, where someone is flogging a book entitled *Why Liberals Suck*.

Sanctimonious Host:
So you're saying that there is something inherently wrong with Liberals.

Book Flogger:
Isn't it obvious Marvin? I mean they are practically a

cancer on the beautiful pure flesh of the thyroid of our nation.

You switch channels again. This time to an infomercial. What's safer than an infomercial? You settle back into your couch and watch as two genetically perfect people who have been surgically altered to smile constantly hold some strange object up for the camera.

Ted:
You know Mary Anne, I can't imagine anything better than making my own homemade Turnip Relishes. With Ted and Mary Anne's patented Turnip Relish Maker!

Mary Anne:
You're right Ted! You'd have to be a moron not to love it!

Ted:
Right, or you'd have to have cancer!

Mary Anne:
Yes, you're right Ted. You'd have to have *cancer*!

Ted:
Yup. Cancer. Cancer Cancer Cancer!

Mary Anne:
Let's make out Ted.

Ted:
I'd love to Mary Anne.

They make out. You pick up the television and hurl it out of your third-storey window killing several harmless squirrels in the process.

OK, I may be exaggerating a little, but it really is fascinating how much the concept of "cancer" is used as a metaphor for the evils of virtually anything in our society. I've heard it used as a comparison to political parties, white collar crime, and yes, even popular sports teams. After receiving your diagnosis, you might be remarkably sensitive to it for a while. It may piss you off, sadden you or (if you have a very different psyche than I do) it might not affect you at all. You might be having a perfectly acceptable day when BAM! Someone will just come up and mention how the current bus drivers' strike is a malignancy on the skin of our fair city. There's not much you can do about it except let it roll off your back as quickly as possible and get on with your day. You might even want to count them up and then say "Hmm. Only four absolutely misplaced cancer references today. Not bad!"

"The world is round and the place which may seem like the end may also be the beginning."
—Ivy Baker Priest

You're Not Going to Be Yourself

A while ago I had a phone conversation with someone who had just found out that she had a malignancy. When she got the news that there was a "little bit of cancer" in her thyroid, she was a bit upset but not that concerned. She went through the next few days and worked like crazy on a number of different projects. A while later, it sunk in. She was doing dishes and cleaning up her apartment when suddenly she burst into tears and couldn't stop crying. Often we hear the news on an intellectual level at a doctor's office or over the phone and feel like we can deal with it very well. We might look "remarkably strong" to everyone and appear to be "bearing up well under the circumstances" but no matter how strong we appear, eventually, this news affects us on a deep psychological and even physical level. You might cry uncontrollably or find yourself in a rage or somewhere in between. The level of intensity the first time you connect with your emotions about this can be a little frightening in itself. Thoughts like "I'm not like this" or "I don't cry like this" are very common while you're having an emotional release. The first time you really feel it might be when you're awake at three in the morning, or home by yourself, or with someone you trust. Heck, it might even happen while you're at the bank machine (if so, people will probably let you go to the front of the line).

The Dam Might Burst

"Grief is itself a medicine"
—**William Cowper Charity**

A huge emotional release that involves tears or anger is perfectly normal right now. In fact, if you aren't ridiculously upset about this at some point, you'd really have something to worry about. Let yourself rage and cry and allow these feelings to flow and get them out of your system. Holding them in (from my experience) can really be detrimental to yourself and those around you.

The one thing to remember even while you're doing this is to keep yourself out of harm's way. Make sure you're in a safe environment and if you're not, go somewhere you know you'll be OK and cry your eyes out.

A Very Healthy Kick in the Stomach

Early in the process for me I was referred to Dr. Andrew Matthew. When I first walked into his office and sat down across from him, I wasn't taking the whole thing seriously. I didn't really *have* cancer at that point, it was just a probability, and besides I was one "Healthy Young Man" and it didn't make sense at all that I would have

15

this strange disease that I figured only smokers and old people who lived next to bauxite mines suffered from. Since I had only lived next to a bauxite mine for a few months, and drank green tea on a regular basis, I thought I was completely in the clear. I walked into Dr. Andrew's office cocky as hell, and sat down.

He looked at me and said very calmly, "So Rob, have you dealt with the fact that this might kill you?" Wow. What a kick in the pants that was. He didn't mince words; he just let me have it right between the eyes. I was remarkably shocked and muttered something about the fact that it was wasn't a sure thing yet. He assured me that, psychologically, it didn't matter. He told me that I was in fight or flight mode already and that I was going to be going through some pretty tough stuff for a while.

What is the Fight or Flight Response?

The fight or flight response goes back an awfully long way in our evolutionary history and we inherited it from our ancestors. When I say ancestors I'm not talking about your great grandfather who made the best moonshine in five counties. No, I'm talking about our common ancestors who were actual reptiles millions and millions of years ago. Fight or flight is a part of our DNA. It is in what is referred to as the reptilian part of our brain and is so embedded in our genetic code that there is no getting rid of it. When we perceive a deadly threat that is external to us, we have one of two immediate instinctive responses. We either get rid of the threat by attacking it or by putting some ground between it and us. This has served us very well over many millennia and subsequently, we have been able to procreate, develop opposable thumbs, and eventually create and watch reality television.

That's All Well and Good, but...

The fight or flight response works fine, except when your good doctor gives you the news about a malignancy in your body. At that moment, these primordial instincts engage in a very big way because a diagnosis of cancer is one of the most threatening pieces of news that you can hear in your entire life, regardless of the actual level of medical risk involved. Consequently, your stress level goes absolutely through the roof. However, with a medical diagnosis, there is nothing external to either fight or run from and as a result your body and psyche have no idea what to do with all of this unused energy that is just coursing through you. You can't physically fight anything. There is no lion attacking you in the middle of the night and there are no bad guys beating down your door. In your current situation what could you possibly attack or run from? Yourself? I can hear you asking right now, "Then what the heck *do* I do Rob?"

Well, I have a few suggestions:

1: Get physical.
Exercise! I found that my desire to beat the living crap out of cab drivers who cut me off on my bike went to a much more manageable level when I was lifting weights and running. Even just thirty minutes a day of physical activity that you enjoy will do you a world of good right now. Walking, running, cycling and yoga did it for me but there are of course, many other physical activities that will help you blow off steam, such as dancing, swimming and even bowling. Essentially, whatever physical activity you enjoy doing, get to it, even if you don't feel like it at the time.

"Melancholy is incompatible with bicycling."
—James E. Starrs

17

2: Write your feelings and thoughts in a journal.

This can be a very useful outlet if you just get your pen moving on the page. Words and then feelings will start to come out, and when they do, it works best if you don't judge them but let them spill. A lot of my journal writing during this period is barely legible printing that is probably still engraved into the table at Starbucks where I wrote it because I was pressing so hard with my pen. I probably ruined three tables this way and am paying Starbucks back by drinking copious amount of lattes.

"Fill your paper with the breathings of your heart."
—William Wordsworth

3: Cry

If you're comfortable with this already, great! You will probably bawl more than once and that is very healthy for you. If this is not comfortable and you're a big tough guy who eats nails for breakfast and flosses with strands of steel wool, well then I've got a question for you: Are you man enough to cry? It takes a really strong person to be that vulnerable. And I'm willing to bet even Chuck Norris cries.

Meanwhile, back at Dr Andrew's office, the good doctor held up an ordinary looking coffee mug and illustrated a very important idea to me. He said that the mug represents our capacity to handle stress in our day-to-day life. Now, the liquid inside that mug represents the actual stress that you are experiencing at any given time. This might be stuff like making a living, being in a relationship, paying your bills etc. The level of the mug might be at a third to half full at any given time. All of this is quite manageable but when a diagnosis of cancer comes into your life, it's the equivalent of pouring three liters of water into this little mug. Of course, water—or stress—spills everywhere and makes a complete mess. When this happens, our ability to handle stress is overloaded and we start acting differently than usual.

In my case, this is putting it mildly. I had bouts of rage that I am not proud of at all. Fortunately, I expressed them in safe ways most of the time. Once, however I managed to yell at a guy at a party. Now, he *was* being a real jerk, but normally I would have handled it in a much different way. I could have told him to get lost like a sane human being or I could have started a frank and useful dialogue about treating people with respect. Instead of doing this, I flipped out. I yelled at him and watched as most of my friends backed away from me while this angry, freaky version of Rob went to town on this poor guy. I didn't hit him, but I really wanted to and it was all I could do to stop. My point is, I was doing something that was *completely* out of character for me and not in a good way. I chalked it up to huge amounts of stress and my pending diagnosis and resolved to be very careful with myself in social situations.

There may be times when emotions run so high for you that writing in your journal is just not going to do it. You may be in a situation where you are close to doing something that is not just out of character, but dangerous. If that happens, you need to manage yourself pretty carefully. Here are a couple of anger management techniques that, although simple, will keep your priceless Ming vase collection intact and also hopefully keep you out of the stockade.

Breathe Deeply and Count to Ten

I know it's been used for centuries, but it works. If you have a burst of anger and you need to control it, breathe deeply and slowly and let the hot rush of feeling drain out of you while you stand in line at the coffee shop. Do this for a slow count to ten and chances are you will have calmed down a bit.

Another thing to do is to leave wherever you are and go somewhere safe immediately. Remove yourself from the situation before you cause some irreparable damage to whatever relationship you're dealing with at the moment. This might be as simple as walking out of the room, or literally stepping back from the conversation in order to regain your composure.

Telling People

"Sometimes the biggest act of courage is a small one."
—Lauren Raffo

Eventually, you're going to have to tell the people that you love (and some people you don't love) that you have this disease. This might seem intimidating, but like many things in life, it gets easier as you go along.

Tell someone whom you trust first.
Sharing this with someone whom you can trust to give you a lot of support is very important. This may be a sibling, grown child, best friend or, if you are lucky enough to have a supportive spouse, it will surely be them. When you first do this, you may be quite upset yourself and there could be tears involved for everyone and that is completely OK.

The best way to tell someone is in a simple and straightforward way. Just take a deep breath and go for it. A useful phrase to start with is "I went to the doctor the other day and..." or "You know I've had some tests done lately? Well I got the results back..." and go on from there. You will probably find that they look at you in shock and then say things like "Oh My God!" They might be so upset that they will start to cry and you will end up comforting and consoling them. This can seem remarkably ironic. I mean, here you are with this big disease and you're telling someone else it's OK? Life can be strange.

After a while, you will get used to the reactions that your family, friends and coworkers have and it may even begin to seem a bit more normal for you.

A Way to Handle This If You Have Young Kids

Our natural instinct with children, of course, is to protect them any way we can. A lot of people's first inclination is to keep knowledge of this disease to themselves and not include the younger members of the family. I understand that completely, but I think it's very important to share with them what's going on with your health. Kids are very intuitive, especially when it concerns the welfare of their parents, so in all likelihood they will know that something is bothering you. It's much better to deal with it up front and include them in your journey in a way that they can understand.

Many parents have found that thinking about telling your kids is often much harder than actually doing it. Tell them in a way that they can understand and is age appropriate. You don't have to explain everything to them all at once. After diagnosis, you might want to tell them that you have something called "cancer" and that you might be sick for a while, but that you're getting really good care from very good doctors. Allow plenty of time for questions when you talk to them and be as honest and straightforward as possible.

As you get closer to different stages of treatment you can explain each event to them. For instance, if you're going to chemo, you might want to explain that you might be tired after you go to the hospital and you might lose your hair for a while. Children can be remarkably resilient and usually have a greater ability to adapt to changing life conditions than we do. Always, of course, let them know that you love them and that one of the best ways to help you feel better is for them to give you lots of hugs.

It's Your Deal

Please be aware that you do not have to tell anyone if you don't want to. You have every right to *not* let everyone know what's up with you. You can even decide exactly who you want to tell and keep it just within your inner circle. If you don't want a lot of fuss, then you can keep it to yourself. You might also want to tell people as a trip to the hospital approaches. Many times there is quite a lengthy gap between the time you get diagnosed and the time you get taken to surgery or begin some kind of treatment. If that's the case, you can keep it quiet until just before the big day and then let everybody know. This might be very handy as it will allow you to deal with all the psychological stuff at your own pace during pre-surgery, and then have everyone's support throughout your physical recovery.

Chapter 3
Battening Down the Hatches

"The healthy and strong individual is the one who asks for help when he needs it."
—**Rona Barrett**

In this chapter:

Why you need a support system
The list on the fridge
Knowing why is crucial
Getting through the toughest times
What to expect during the identity shuffle
Forgive yourself if you're off kilter

One very remarkable trait we humans have is our ability to get used to virtually anything. The day a plane crashes in your backyard, you might be pretty freaked out about it, but in a week or so, it will just seem like part of life to have the FAA sifting through wreckage while you sip coffee on the porch. No matter how traumatic hearing about this health event is, in time you will get used to it. You might find that even in a week or two you will be, on some level, able to accept your new circumstances. After you've gotten over the initial shock of your diagnosis, and realized you still are who you are, albeit with a significant challenge in your life, there are a few simple things you can do to make this easier.

Set Up Your Support System

Once you've told people, a useful thing to do is get a list of folks you trust who you can call or talk to at anytime. When you wake up at 3 AM having some really scary thoughts and not feeling particularly healthy in spirit, it's great to know that you can speak to someone who cares about you. This could be your spouse, close friend, a grown child, or it might even be a "helpline" for people in distress.

So get yourself a list of three to five folks who you can call anytime. Here's how to set it up in advance. Over a coffee or the next time you're on the phone with someone you want to be on your list, say something like this:

"Hey, I could really use a favour."
"Sure what's up?"
"Well, you know I'm going through cancer treatment right now."
"God yes....I am so sorry. If there's anything I can do…"
"Funny you should ask, because there is."
"Name it!"
"There may be some times when I'm scared or upset and I'm going to need somebody to talk to. So I was wondering if I could have an arrangement with you where I could call you night or day if I really need a friend and you would just talk to me."
"Of course!"
"I'm doing OK now but there might be times when I really need a friend."
"I'd be honoured!"

See? Not that hard…

If you have a spouse and you want to talk to them, you can set it up in much the same way…

"Hey, sweetie, you know I'm pretty worried these days."
"Of course."
"Well, sometimes I might wake up in the middle of the night and need your help."
"Sure."
"If I wake up and can't get back to sleep, is it OK if I wake you so you can sit with me?"
"Absolutely!"

Just like that. I know this might seem obvious and simple but it is also very important. There were many times when I needed to talk to somebody at 4 AM but didn't, because I didn't want to disturb their sleep. So instead, I watched infomercials and spent my retirement fund on "revolutionary" new pasta makers and seminars like "The 7 Grain Real Estate Solution." I would have been much better off talking to a friend. If you arrange this beforehand, you are much more likely to seek their help when you need it. Keep this list of folks somewhere handy so that if the time comes, it will be there for you.

The List on the Fridge

Another strategy to help you through difficult days is to make yourself a list of things that you really like to do. On days when you're not feeling very well and you are really wallowing in fear or depression (this can definitely happen, BTW) go to your list and do something that will help you feel a lot better.

A Possible List on the Fridge
1: Go for a walk in the park.
2: Take yourself to a movie.

3: Get your spouse to take you out to lunch.

4: Make a list of places you want to go in the world.

5: Donate some extra clothes to charity.

6: Give some money to a homeless person on the street.

7: Put on your favourite comedy DVD and laugh your ass off.

8: Crank call a teacher from high school who pissed you off.

9: Get a massage.

10: Dance to music you love for ten minutes.

Give yourself at least ten of these possibilities and on days when it's really tough, you can just call out a number from one to ten when you're in bed, and go and find out which one you've chosen and then do it.

The Big "Why"

"He who has a why to live can bear almost any how."
—**Friedrich Nietzsche**

It's also very important to know why you are going to get through this. Personally, I knew that I really wanted to share useful information with people about this experience, and that if there was any way for me to make this easier for folks then I was going to do it. I also realized that I really wanted to be around the people I love, and knew I would fight like hell to be able to stay with them. A third "why" for me was the fact that there were (and are) many parts of the world that I haven't visited yet. Knowing these "whys" was enough to keep me in the game and keep me committed to getting healthy again. So think of your whys and write them down.

In fact you might want to write them down now...

Why am I going to get through this?

1: People I love who I need to spend time with (list five)

2: Things I haven't done yet and would really love to (list five)

3: Things I already love that I will do after I recover (list five)

The most challenging time of day for me was 4 AM. Reason and hope were nowhere to be found at that dark hour and I would wake up, swear at my doctor, go to my fridge, and then watch reruns of M*A*S*H* until I finally fell back to sleep on my couch at five thirty. If I had any advice to give you for your particular 4 AM (your particular 4 AM might be in the afternoon) it would be first of all, to realize that you will feel better in the morning or at some point the next day. Funnily enough, four or five in the morning is when our bodies are at their lowest ebb. We are trying to rest and regenerate at a very deep level and our circadian rhythms are at their absolute nadir during this point in our daily cycle. So if you run into Despair in the middle of the night, please remember that the time of day probably has something to do with it.

I think there are two ways you can deal with the four-in-the-morning blues. You can either: **1) Distract yourself** or **2) Really feel the feelings**.

#1) Distract yourself
You might want to prep for this. Have a couple of videos around that you really like, Grab something light and funny and *not* something they would study at the NYU

film program. *Anchorman* and *Austin Powers* are perfect at 4 AM. If you paint, put on some gentle music and paint. Paint ugly angry pictures or really calm gentle ones. Have a book around that will really take your mind of things. Essentially, whatever you like to do that is gentle and easy for you will help you get through these tricky wee hours. Sometimes even going from your bed to your couch and trying to sleep there will help you nod off.

#2) Really feel the feelings.
Many times during the day we have our emotional survival gear on in a very big way. This is necessary in order to get through work, pay the bills, and ride the bus with a bunch of strangers. When we have a diagnosis of cancer kicking around in our psyche, we tend to double up on our armor and really gird our loins, otherwise we'd never be able to get through anything. That's why our family, friends and coworkers look at us and say, "Wow, you're dealing with it so well!" or "You're so strong!" Meanwhile we fall apart when we're alone. How does this relate to four in the morning? Well, when there is no one around, we have very little reason to "be strong for someone else." Thus, this is really prime time to get all the bad emotional stuff out. So, let yourself cry, or scream into a pillow. You will get rid of a lot of bad stuff and might even tire yourself out enough to sleep.

A special note to guys: I'm a six-foot, 200 hundred pound, poker playing bastard and I bawled like a baby. It's okay. It really is. (And I was still a six-foot, 200 hundred pound, poker playing bastard the next day.)

When It's Darkest

"If you're going through hell, keep going."
—Winston Churchill

Alright, we have to talk about this. I hate to admit it, but I occasionally had suicidal feelings at this time of the day. I never got to the point where I was really in danger, but there were a couple times when my emotions got the best of me and things got a bit scary. You have to do some pretty good self-management at these times. If you really feel like you're going to do something to hurt yourself, then it is time to *get out your list of family and friends* whom you can call at any time. You may have already said to them, "I might call you in the middle of the night because I need to talk to someone." You have the rest of your life to take them out to lunch to make up for it. Think about how pissed they'll be if you don't ask for their help. So if you get to this point, pick up the phone and call someone.

Doing the Identity Shuffle

Your identity may get a bit of a shake-up after you are diagnosed. We are constantly walking around in the world with this thing called a self-image which gives us a sense of who we are in relation to our friends, family, salesmen, and the rest of the world. Our sense of self, represented by a list of characteristics in a descending order of importance might go something like this:

Rob
Son
Lover
Actor
Writer
Proud Uncle
Cyclist
Poker player
Man who doesn't clean his kitchen enough

You get the idea. The stuff at the top of the list is more

basic to us. It is in fact what we consider to be at the core of who we are and how we relate ourselves to the rest of the world. Somebody else's might go like this:

Jessica
Mom
Sister
Friend
Actuarial Accountant
Brilliant chef who specializes in seafood

When you get a diagnosis of cancer, this list of characteristics that you hold as your identity gets shaken up in a very big way and all of a sudden, instead of your primary family relationships or your profession being at the top of the list, it might look something more like this.

Rob
Person with cancer
Son
Proud Uncle
Actor
Writer
Guy who wakes up at three in the morning
Owner of several revolutionary pasta makers

As you can see, a new entry to your list has gone screaming to the top. Last week it was nowhere to be found but all of a sudden it has come out of nowhere like the Beatles in 1964 (yes, I'm over forty). Like the Beatles, this new thing that has hit the top of your personal identity chart changes everything. You need time to get through this and adjust to the idea of it. Once you get started making this adjustment, you might find that every conversation you have relates to the fact that you have this condition called cancer.

For instance:
It's a rainy Tuesday afternoon at a bustling accounting

firm. The Boss walks into your office.

Boss:
Henderson, I really need that file on the Quimbery account in the next hour. Will it be ready?

You:
Ram the Quimbery file up your ass, Boss. I've got cancer!

Let's take another example:
It's a chilly morning in December in a major urban center. A bus comes to a stop on Dufferin Street just south of Dundas. The driver opens the door and a line of folks file on trying to get to their accounting firm so they can work on the Quimbery file (that's one big file):

Bus Driver:
That'll be $2.75 please.

You:
How can you ask for a fare when I've got cancer!

You get the idea. This is going to be front and center for a while and its going to take up a lot of your conscious thoughts and feelings. Hopefully you have a bunch of very understanding people around you who will just let you talk it out.

But if you're not going to be yourself then who are you going to be? Are you going to be the crazy guy who stands at your street corner and goes on about Ancient Sumarian Glass Blowing? Probably not. Will you be Wayne Gretzky, the greatest hockey player of all time? Not unless you started out as Gretzky (and if you're Gretzky and you're reading this book, sorry you've got the Big C. You'll crush it like you crushed one hundred points in a season). My guess is you'll be a more confused, angrier, sadder version of yourself. There will be many times when you will say to yourself "That's not

31

like me!" This again, is normal and you should really cut yourself a lot of slack and know that when you recover you will feel much more like yourself, but for now, you're in for a bit of a ride.

Where the heck is God?

It is quite possible that your feelings about the Creator may take a bit of a hit in the next while. They certainly did in my case. At the time, I felt kind of bad about it. I mean what's worse than cursing God? Won't He be striking me down anytime now? Isn't that a lightning bolt heading straight for my apartment? After a while though, I decided that if there actually is a God, She is probably tough enough to take my little bit of anger directed His way. And, if She is a loving, forgiving being (unlike my grade seven shop teacher), then He probably won't mind that I rail at Her a bit and (God forbid) take His name in vain. It just seems that if God is all powerful, loving and created us in Her image then I think He can take the fact that we're pissed off. I mean really pissed off. So go ahead. God can take it.

Throughout the first part of this journey, you will probably be initially shocked by your condition and adjusting your psyche and spirit to what lies ahead. This takes a great deal of patience and forgiveness for yourself and your behaviours. It's useful to allow yourself a lot of leeway in terms of what you need at any given time. You might be fine one minute and able to deal with whatever is facing you, and the next minute you might burst into tears. All of this is par for the course. Let it happen, but let it happen *safely*. There is a big difference between releasing emotion in a way that helps you and carrying on in a way that could hurt you and those you love. So give yourself the space to do this in a healthy way.

If there is any good news in this chapter at all, and I'd like to think that there is, it's that the "you" that you were before this, will still exist. You might change a bit; you might even wind up stronger for the experience. You might tend to take less crap or you might let trivial things that used to bother you roll off your back, but you will still be yourself. You've got a whole lot of life in front of you and a ton to give, so hang in there. Meanwhile, we have some things to talk about...

Chapter 4
Getting Yourself Educated

In this chapter:

What is cancer anyway?
How are cancers different?
How to talk to your doctor
What about statistics?
Finding a community
Great Web resources
Should I go down the naturopathy route?

Getting yourself educated helps for a few reasons. For one, you feel like you are doing something (because you are) and also you are giving yourself more resources and finding out what the road ahead can bring. This will help you tremendously in feeling like you have some power and choice in the situation. As my good friend Dr. Matthew said to me, "You're going to have to kick some ass on this one."

When I got my diagnosis of cancer (or probable cancer), I was shocked. My first impulse was to completely freeze up and not do anything at all. Heck, I'll admit that I was the proverbial bunny in the headlights. It can be such a shock that all you want to do is sit in your "hidey hole" and not come out for a while, which is exactly what I did until I walked into Dr. Matthew's office. He looked me square in the eyes and said "Rob, you've got to learn what's going on and go into this with your eyes wide open." I didn't want to learn about what my condition was, but once I began it got a lot easier and made every part of the journey better.

We've all heard the word a hundred times a week, at least. But what exactly *is* cancer? Well, put very simply, cancer is growth that is out of control. It is the unrestricted reproduction of cells in an unhealthy way. Of course, cells have to reproduce all the time in order for your body to renew itself; in fact, the cells in our body renew themselves at different rates depending on their function and place in the body. For instance, the cells in the stomach lining reproduce every 7-10 days while some other cells in the body can live for many years. All of that is fine, but sometimes this growth gets out of hand and cells reproduce at a rate that the body cannot handle.

Cancer cells develop because of damage to DNA. DNA is in every cell and directs all of the cell's activities. Most of the time when DNA becomes damaged, either the cell dies or it is able to repair the DNA. In cancer cells, the damaged DNA is not repaired.

How is Cancer like Donald Trump?

Let's bring an analogy to this. You probably know what it's like to walk or drive down a street almost every day for years. Then, seemingly overnight, what was a vacant lot with some trees and grass becomes a condo development with a name like "Pretentious Towers." Then a while later, you see a condo called "Sterling Vista, An Exclusive Adult Lifestyle Community, Now with Bowling!" and after that a cute little concrete slab called "You Wish You Could Live Here! Residences for the Rude and Annoying!" Before you know it, what was once a nice, calm neighborhood is awash in overpriced 400 square-foot apartments that sell for $750,000 each. How is this like cancer? Well, cancer is growth that is unsustainable and harmful to the larger organism itself, while normal growth takes into account the health of the entire living being. Cancer in a nutshell, could be called "greedy growth."

How Cancers Differ

Cancers can begin in many different parts of the body. But different types of cancer can act very differently. For example, lung cancer and breast cancer are very different diseases. They grow at different rates and respond to different treatments. That's why people with cancer need treatment that is aimed at their particular variety of the disease.

How Cancer Spreads

Cancer usually forms as a tumor (a lump or mass). Some cancers, like leukemia, do not form tumors. Instead, these cancer cells involve the blood and blood-forming organs, and circulate through other tissues where they grow.

Cancer cells often travel through the bloodstream or through the lymph system to other parts of the body where they begin to grow and replace normal tissue. This spreading process is called *metastasis*.

Even when cancer has spread to a different part of the body it is still named for the place in the body where it started. For example, breast cancer that has spread to the liver is metastatic breast cancer, not liver cancer. Prostate cancer that has spread to the bone is called metastatic prostate cancer, not bone cancer.

Remember that not all tumors are cancerous. *Benign* (non-cancerous) tumors do not spread to other parts of the body (metastasize) and are very rarely life-threatening.

How Common is Cancer?

Half of all men and one-third of all women in the US and Canada will develop this disease during their lifetimes. Probably more people get cancer than watch "Family Guy" reruns. Today, millions of people are living with cancer or have had it. The risk of developing most types of this disease can sometimes be reduced by changes in a person's lifestyle; for example, by quitting smoking, limiting time in the sun, being physically active, and having a better diet.

How to Talk to Your Doctor

When sitting in your doctor's office, it can be challenging to keep your train of thought. I found that my usual confident manner went out the window when I was speaking about this with the numerous specialists I went to. It was very useful to have a notebook with questions written down so I could just refer to them and read them off my list.

Some possible questions for your doctor:
In your opinion, what is the percentage chance that I have cancer?
What is the course of treatment for this?
How long will this course of treatment take?

Can you give me an indication of my chances of recovery?
How will my lifestyle change after I recover?
What can I do now to help the healing process?
Can you suggest any resources (local support groups) that would be useful for me?

Write the answers down, even in very short point form because what may seem crystal clear in the doctor's office can slip your mind once you leave. Worse yet, your imagination can take over and you can exaggerate what you've heard. If a doctor says "You've got a 10% chance of malignancy," your overactive mind could morph it into "Your kidney is about to explode!" I found it very useful to repeat things back to my doctor, just to make sure I was getting the information right. I'd say "I have to repeat this back, because I'm a bit freaked out and I want to make sure I'm getting this right. You're saying that…" and then I'd repeat what he had told me. This worked very well with doctors who were patient (pun!) as I could really make sure I was getting it right the first time.

Your doctor may be terrific at helping you get educated. He or she may be a regular font of generosity and knowledge. Or not. The reality of many health care systems is that doctors have very narrow windows of time for each appointment, so their allotted time to give you a life-altering diagnosis may be only fifteen minutes. Because of that, they may rush you a bit, but feel free to slow them down and say "I really need to have you just answer a couple of questions for me," and go from there. If you don't find out everything you need, there are many more resources at your disposal that you can utilize as well.

Newsflash: Your Doctor May Be Human!

I was raised to respect authority. I'm guessing that most of you were as well. Now, one of the groups of people who have a *ton* of authority and respect in our society are people with MDs after their name. When we have this crazy diagnosis floating around in our lives, and we go to the doctor we tend to treat everything that the Doc says as sacrosanct (I'm really just thrilled to put the word "sacrosanct" in a sentence.) We think it is remarkably impertinent (OK, maybe "impertinent" is pushing it) for us to even question the doctor on anything at all. Well, it's time to get over that quickly.

I'm all for doctors. In fact, a couple have saved my life. However, I have noticed that doctors are actually human beings. This means that they can make mistakes, they sometimes don't know everything about a subject, and they don't necessarily have the time to read absolutely all of the research that relates to your specific case. With that in mind, it's really useful to look at your doctor as a great and terrific resource in your journey back to health. He or she is not the only way back, nor does he/she have all the answers. *You* are the most important caregiver you will ever have. You are running the show and you need to know what's going on. This will radically change how you feel about healing and help you switch from feeling like a victim to feeling and acting like the capable and powerful person you are. You are your own best resource at this point. But don't worry, you're not going through this alone: you have many more resources than you think and many people around who can help.

Survivors

People who have gone through this already can be a great resource for you. There are many survivors around you right now who have beaten this already and who can tell you what it was like for them and what to expect. The super in your building may have dealt with a bout of the big C a few years ago. Or you may find out that a friend's brother has gone through virtually the same thing as you. These folks will have strategies that they can share with you about how to best get through it.

"85% of statistics are made up on the spot."
—Todd Snider, country singer

Study Up

I think statistics are very useful as long as they serve you. I have a friend who intentionally avoided the statistics about her condition. She didn't want to know what the survival rates were or what her odds were for a full recovery, and it served her. In my own experience, I came down with thyroid cancer at 40. Now, as an otherwise very healthy young (humour me…) man the odds of that happening were very low. Really low. However, it happened. In fact it was so weird that my doctors kept looking at me and saying. "Are you sure you didn't live next to a leaking nuclear reactor?" The point is the stats would suggest that I wasn't going to get this diagnosis, but I did.

So, here's what I suggest with stats: if they say you have an 85% chance of full recovery, brilliant! Statistics are amazing! You are going to get through it. If they say you have a 15% chance of making it through then, damn it, you're going to be part of the 15%. You may think this is a bit self-delusional but be aware that you have to play some mental games with yourself during this time.

A great way to get educated is to use the library. It's free. Its sitting right there in your neighbourhood with a gazillion books on virtually whatever you want. You can also order stuff in from other libraries to your local branch. I know this isn't rocket science in any way but many folks overlook the easiest and best resources that they have right in front of them. This is a treasure trove at your complete disposal.

Go to a Group

One of the biggest challenges common to people going through treatment is a sense of isolation and aloneness. You might need some allies and friends who know something about your journey. Where do you get this? From a support group. It is a very useful thing to have a group of folks who you can talk to (or even just listen to) who are going through the same thing. This will give you very valuable human contact and really help you feel connected to the world around you. There will be people in different stages of treatment as well and you can compare notes on different doctors and treatments. But really, the most profound experience you will get with a group will be your sense of connection to other people who are going through the same thing. People will sit in a circle and talk, and you will know that *you are not alone*.

It should be fairly easy to find a support group in your community. Just Google your community's name and "Cancer Support Group" and this should get you started.

You may be lucky enough to live in a community with a Gilda's Club. Gilda's has over 20 clubhouses in the US and Canada where people living with cancer and their families can go for community support and education.

If you live near a Gilda's, I highly recommend that you drop in. Explain your situation and they will tell you about all the resources that they offer for free. No matter where you are, you can find a community. Look online or ask your doctor for a list of resources to get you started finding a community that can help you out.

There are many more resources for folks going through cancer now than there were even a few years ago. You could ask your receptionist at your doctor's office if she can suggest anything. I must admit, I felt alone through a lot of this, but I realize now that I didn't need to at all. There were many more resources around me that would have been tremendously helpful, but at the time I was shy to ask for help, or didn't even know where to begin. All I had to do was reach out in any direction and the journey would have been much easier. I hope you give yourself the gift of asking for help. It's out there and will do you a world of good.

The Web: Treasure Chest or Bucket of Crap?

We live in a world where any person with access to Google can find out virtually anything. What's the average annual rainfall in the Gobi desert? (about 194 mm a year). What was the earth's population in the year 1 AD? (about 300 million). I found out these fascinating facts in about one minute. Today, any ten year old can do research that would have a scholar thirty years ago tearing the patches off of his elbows in envy. A huge chunk of the world's knowledge is at our fingertips, and this is terrific for those of us in our situation.

The Web is potentially a good resource, but you've got to be very careful when using it. The great thing about the Web is that anybody can publish anything. The bad thing about the Web is that anybody can publish anything. There is terrific, well-researched information and there is some absolute garbage that could prove dangerous. The trick is to be very careful about what you take seriously, especially with something as important as your health.

Great Web Resources

Having said all that, here are some terrific Web resources that you might find useful. The Web is terrific at community-building and bringing folks together to share information and support. Here are some sites that can help you with both:

**Cancer Buddies Network
(www.cancerbuddiesnetwork.org)**
A place for people with cancer to connect and share stories and information on getting through cancer.

**The National Coalition For Cancer Survivorship
(www.canceradvocacy.org)**
A terrific site with many resources for survivors.

**Cancer Support Community
(www.thewellnesscommunity.org)**
A site with global outreach for people going through cancer and their families.

Planet Cancer (www.planetcancer.org)
Online support for teens and young adults. Excellent information and community connection in a positive atmosphere complete with a dose of comic irreverence.

Any of these sites will get you started in getting you more educated about your condition. As well, you will see that there are many other folks in the world just like you who are getting through this one day at a time. If I had had access to these resources, my own journey would have been so much easier. Instead of reaching out, or even asking for help, I chose to stay isolated and this made my journey much harder than it needed to be. At the time, I thought this proved that I was tough and made me more of a man. I was wrong. I urge you to reach out, either online or in your local community, and to connect with people going through similar journeys.

Should I Go down the Naturopathy Route?

In my very humble opinion, Western medicine has a pickle up its own butt. I realize that doctors do remarkable things. Yes, they saved my life and yes, I am very happy about that. However, every time I mentioned any kind of alternative therapy to a medical doctor I was hushed up like an errant twelve-year-old. My naturopath, a doctor whom I respect very much, was giving me care at the same time that I was being treated by traditional doctors.

Dr. Kim (the naturopath) was thorough and very effective in his treatment of me. He listened, counseled and gave me very good care. When I mentioned to my traditional doctor that I was seeing a naturopath, he looked at me with great alarm and said "This is cancer. No amount of massage is going to make it go away." I hadn't mentioned massage at all. He just assumed that seeing a naturopath would involve working with massage. I mentioned this to Dr. Kim later and he was remarkably unsurprised. He explained it like this: "The vast majority of traditional doctors are completely threatened by naturopathy or virtually any type of treatment that does not fit into their very strict ideas of what medicine, that is, Western medicine, is."

This is interesting, considering Dr. Kim had helped me with many problems in the past and was able to diagnose and treat me for things that left my more traditional doctors scratching their heads. I'm not saying to run out and get yourself a bag of chicken bones and wave them over yourself three times a day, but I am saying though that there are so-called nontraditional methods of treatment that have been around for a long time that can give you tremendous benefits. Specifically, naturopathic medicine and acupuncture practiced by licensed professionals can help you heal faster and reduce your level of discomfort. If you do choose to integrate these treatments with Western medicine, make sure that the different methods of healing do not interfere with each other and thereby reduce their effectiveness. Inform your medical doctor that you are seeking alternative therapy. I found the careful integration of different treatments very useful, and in some instances (specifically with post-surgical recovery), I found a gifted naturopath to be a godsend.

During this time, you will probably be thinking about your condition almost every waking moment. As a result, you may find that unexpected resources may seemingly drop out of the sky. All you will have to do is pay attention and follow the leads that the world provides. You can call this synchronicity (thanks Carl Jung!), or you might think that it's mere coincidence, but you will notice that resources will just appear right in front of you. It might be a book leant by a coworker or a conversation with a bus driver that gives you a valuable insight; or you might run into an old friend after a long time of not seeing them.

I think that when we're going through a challenging time, we are led down a path or shown markers along the way that will make our journey a bit easier. Call it otherworldly guidance or whatever you like, but I was aware that when I was sick I had some mysterious coincidences occur that were downright uncanny. Whether this was a nod from a higher source or not didn't really matter to me, because in this situation, we can use all the help we can get.

What's That around the Next Bend?

Getting yourself educated does two essential things for you. First, it lets you know what you'll likely experience next. Second, it changes your role from that of a passive victim to someone who is taking control of his life and his situation. The faster you can feel like you have some kind of influence in your life and that you are not merely at the mercy of your condition, the better off you will be.

You will also be more relaxed and more able to use the resources that are around you. If you are in a horrible, fearful state, then your chances of using what you have are very low. With knowledge of your condition, you give yourself a flashlight to shine on your self-doubt and fear, and this will take away a lot of the panic that initially comes with having a diagnosis.

This gives you a great advantage in dealing with your situation because you know what to expect with your condition. It gives you the power to know what your chances of a full recovery are and it helps you to know how long it will take you to get back to your life again.

Chapter 5
Testing... Testing...

"Smooth seas do not make skillful sailors."
—**African Proverb**

In this chapter:

The waiting room
Bring an ally
What are these tests anyway?
What to expect from common treatments
Navigating the medical profession
You are your own best advocate

There are very few certainties in life, but one thing I am sure of is that there are many tests involved in getting treatment for cancer. There will be biopsies and ultrasounds and then ultrasounds to confirm the results of the biopsy. After a while, you will think that you are finally finished being poked, prodded, and scanned; then your doctor will advise you to undergo a few more tests just to be sure. It was surprising to me that I found these tests a bit unsettling. After all, they're just tests, so what's the big deal?

The one saving grace is that you can't stay up all night

studying for an MRI. Even though we can't cram for these examinations like we did back in school, it's good to know some things about them beforehand so it will be less of an ordeal when you go in. You might think "Hey, I'm just going in for a biopsy, this should be a breeze!" but your psyche can't be fooled that easily and it knows that something is up regardless of what you tell it. There are some challenges during this period, but of course there are also strategies to help get you through this with your psyche and spirit intact.

Someone found it convenient to put all the nervous people waiting for a test in the same place and call it, quite obviously, "The Waiting Room." When you go to an appointment there will be a bunch of people there, all of whom will be as uncomfortable as you. In fact, remember that first high school dance in your home town, when the girl you had a crush on was flirting with Brock from the wrestling team and you just stood with your back against the wall and didn't dance all night because you were scared and you thought everyone was having a good time except you? No? Well, maybe that was just me. The point is probably everyone was uncomfortable to a certain degree (even Brock, who now runs a failing hardware store.) Waiting rooms are a lot like this, simply because we are all experts at looking like we're fine when actually we're remarkably nervous. So, when you are sitting and waiting for your name to be called, look around the room at all the supposedly composed people and remember that they are as freaked out as you are.

That's the first thing to do. The second thing to do is breathe. Breathe slowly and deeply. If you feel yourself getting a bit nervous, just take in a long slow breath, hold it for a few seconds and then release it. Do this a few times and your body will get the message.

You're going to need a distraction or two while you're

waiting for your tests. Bring things with you that will help you pass the time and give you comfort. I'm all for getting educated but I don't think the waiting room is the place to read medical information. Grab a trashy novel or a book of humour to help you through it; otherwise you'll be staring at the December issue of *Weights and Measures* magazine. You might want to bring along an MP3 player whenever you can and select a playlist that relaxes you. Music can really wash away anxiety and make the whole situation a lot more bearable. I'm a fan of Eddie Izzard's stand up, so I would listen to that whenever I was scared and it really helped. Gentle classical music, a book on tape or even a recording of ocean waves can be very soothing to listen to while you wait.

It's a great idea to bring a notebook to your appointments. This can be used to write down any questions you think of during the test so that you can bring them up with your doctor later.

The Mighty Receptionist

We all know that in the world of medical health, doctors are at the top of the food chain. However, I noticed when I was in my surgeon's office that the doctors may be the kings and queens of their domain but the receptionists hold the keys to that kingdom by controlling the all-powerful appointment book.

I was seeing my surgeon for a pre-op examination and he said that he needed to see me again in six weeks. Like a good patient, I told this to the receptionist and she responded with "That's impossible, he's booked up solid for at least two months. I can maybe get you in, in about nine weeks or so."

"But he said I should get in at about 6 weeks."

"I know sir, but really it's just a few weeks after that. It'll be OK."

It surprised me that she had so much power over the doctor's time and subsequently my medical care. The difference in time turned out to be no big deal, but it really illustrated to me that the person outside the doctor's office with the appointment book has a lot of power. My advice: be very, very nice to them. Get to know their name, chat with them a bit and just generally be a decent person around them.

Bring an Ally!

Having an ally accompany you on these trips can be a big help. This could be your lover, your buddy, your sister, your father, your daughter, your best pal from high school or someone else whom you trust, but whoever it is, they will help you tremendously in dealing with the stress of the dreaded test. They should be someone you are very comfortable with, someone who is calm and can offer you support. If you're a bit nervous about asking them and don't want to be a pain, just reverse the situation and ask yourself this question, "If they were staring down a medical examination and were nervous about it, would I want to go with them?" Of course you would! You're a supportive person and so are they, so give them a chance to show it.

You can do this very simply by saying something like "Hey Buella, I'm going off to a biopsy tomorrow and I'm a bit nervous about it, would you mind coming with me?" Done. If they balk or say they can't, then ask someone else. Some folks are so uncomfortable with hospitals and any hint of mortality that they won't be able to handle doing this. If that's the case, you can go on your own.

A Brief Guide to Tests

"We have two options, medically and emotionally: give up, or fight like hell."
—**Lance Armstrong**

Ultrasound

The ultrasound is a very commonly used method of making a medical diagnosis. It is non invasive (no needles!) and is completely painless. During an ultrasound, sound waves that cannot be heard by the human ear are projected from a wand onto your body and an electronic image is produced that the ultrasound technician records. This is then given to your doctor who somehow interprets the black and white squiggles and from this they can get a closer "look" inside your body. The only mildly uncomfortable part about this is the lubricant they place on you during the examination. This is really no big deal, although I always thought that anytime somebody puts lubricant on me, I expect to have a much better time and be bought dinner beforehand.

The Biopsy

During a biopsy, a medical professional will take a syringe that is a bit wider than the kind they give you the flu shot with and insert it into their area of interest. They then take a small sample of your growth and remove it from your body. They might shift the syringe slightly while it's in your growth in order to get tissue from different sections of the lump. This will give them a better sample and will help them make a more thorough diagnosis. I'm not gonna lie, this hurt a bit. In my case, it hurt not as much as stubbing my toe, but more than learning that Sidney Crosby was going to play for the Penguins. So really, the biopsy is not the piece of cake

51

that the ultrasound is, but it will be over before you know it.

The sample they take is then sent down to the lab where they work up the pathology on the bit of tissue, which simply means that they can actually examine the cells themselves for signs of malignancy.

Endoscopy

A gastrointestinal endoscope is a flexible tube with a tiny camera on the end that is inserted into the anus, in order to view the digestive tract. This test could hardly be described as comfortable, but you may be given mild sedation if your medical professional deems it necessary. This test is used to look for abnormalities in the digestive tract, especially as a screen for colorectal cancers.

MRI

MRI stands for Magnetic Resonance Imaging. This is a painless test that utilizes a magnetic field and radio frequency sound waves to make images of the body. During the test, the patient is placed within a chamber surrounded by a magnetic field. This examination can take up to an hour and does take place in an enclosed area, so if you are sensitive to tight spaces (as I am) then this may take a bit of patience to get through. However, this is a painless procedure and completely non-invasive.

Mammogram

A mammogram uses low-dose radiation to detect breast cancer in women. The breast is compressed and X-rays are used to create an image of the body. Mammograms are used in the early detection and screening of breast cancer and are particularly useful because they can detect minute changes in the breast tissue over a number of years, long before a woman could feel them herself. This is an uncomfortable procedure and should not be done a week before a woman's period, if at all possible, because of the sensitivity experienced during that time.

Decompression

OK, let's say it: tests suck! I hated going for tests. Its not that they were painful, it's just that they can really bring to light the reality of the situation. It can be a bit like walking down the street and feeling like everything is fine and then having someone jump out from behind a recycling bin and hit you in the face with a ten-pound bass. So even though you think "Hey that didn't hurt at all, I'll just go right back to work" you might be taken aback and a bit more upset than you thought.

When you have a test or an appointment with a doctor it's very useful to reserve yourself a window of time afterwards so you can process what happened before you get on with your day. I realize that you're running the UN and you must get back immediately, but in all probability the world will not fall apart if you take another half hour to adjust to what just happened. Even if it's a simple ultrasound that is completely painless and you feel fine, it's OK to let the Trade Minister from Paraguay just cool his jets for awhile. Go and get yourself a coffee or herbal tea and just sit there for a few minutes. You might want to write something in your trusty notebook. Another great thing to do is to call your spouse, family member or close friend to just check in about what happened—they'll probably want to know. During the conversation, you might find out that you have more feelings about this test than you thought. You might feel fine at first, but once you start speaking, all kinds of things might start rolling out of you. Anger at the test itself, how funny/irritating the technician was or how hot the patient across from you was in their tight Flamenco pants: whatever you're feeling, let it settle before you get on your horse and ride into the world again.

"The miracle is not to fly in the air, or to walk on the water, but to walk on the earth."
—**Chinese Proverb**

A Brief Look at Common Treatments

One of the things Dr. Matthew (remember him?) told me in his office so long ago was that even with all the fancy technology and many treatments available to medical practitioners, the only options in treating cancer come down to these three words: cut, burn, and poison. Within these three options, of course there are many different types of treatment and many kinds of surgery but they still come down to these three things.

1: Surgery
Surgery as a treatment for cancer is quite easy to understand. A surgeon physically removes all of the cancerous tissue from the patient. It is common for the surgical team to remove some healthy tissue around the malignant area to ensure that all of the cancer is eliminated (www.mayoclinic.com). There are many types of cancer surgery, including cryosurgery (which involves the use of cold materials like liquid nitrogen to freeze cancer cells), laser surgery (which utilizes beams of high energy light to vaporize or shrink the cancer) and laparoscopic surgery (which involves a small incision in the body and the use of a tiny camera with surgical tools to get rid of the cancer and avoid a large incision).

What's it like to have cancer surgery?
Surgeries for cancer differ widely depending on where the malignancy is and how invasive the procedure needs to be. Some take hours and require more than one night in the hospital before a patient can go home, while others

are actually outpatient surgeries that allow a person to go home and sleep in his or her own bed.

Side Effects
If a general anesthetic is used during the procedure, then the patient will experience a feeling of grogginess and weakness after surgery. Pain associated with the procedure is managed by intravenous meds like morphine and painkillers, like Tylenol 3, which contain codeine.

2: Radiation Therapy (or Radiotherapy)
Radiation Therapy uses X-rays and other forms of radiation (such as gamma rays) to treat the disease. Cells in the treated area have their DNA damaged by the radiation and then it is impossible for them to grow and multiply. Radiation therapy can be used to increase the chances that cancer will not come back after surgery; it is even a cure for some cancers.

What is radiation therapy like?
Most radiation therapy is administered externally. What this means is that a patient usually does not have to stay overnight and will go in for several treatments over a period of 2-8 weeks for five days a week. The medical professional giving the treatment will makes sure the patient is in a proper position by arranging him on a large table or flat surface. Once prepared, the technician will leave the radiation room in much the same way that a dentist leaves the room when someone gets an X-ray. The treatment itself is painless, usually takes only a few minutes and when the patient leaves the hospital they can interact normally with family and friends (National Cancer Institute Website).

Side Effects
This form of cancer treatment, although not painful in itself, has side effects that can include hair loss, fatigue, nausea and skin damage. The length and intensity of the

side effects vary according to a patient's age, the strength of the treatment and where the cancer is located.

3: Chemotherapy

Chemotherapy involves the use of anti-cancer drugs (called cytotoxic drugs) to kill cancer cells. There are at least 50 chemotherapy drugs and often more than one is administered at a time in something that is called "combination chemotherapy" (www.CancerBackup.org). Chemotherapy can be administered a number of ways including orally, through a muscle injection, or intravenously. Chemotherapy is commonly used in conjunction with other cancer therapies.

What is chemotherapy like?

Chemotherapy is administered at a hospital or cancer treatment center. The patient can be given the drugs by taking a pill, getting an intravenous drip, or by injection. Some patients report feeling numbness, burning and tingling during treatment. Chemotherapy is usually given in a cycle. A patient might get chemo everyday for a specific number of days or weeks. These treatments can be followed by a rest period so the healthy cells can heal. The treatment schedule may be repeated for several months (Canadian Cancer Society Website, National Cancer Institute).

Side Effects

During treatment, chemotherapy can also harm healthy cells, which may cause side effects like hair loss, anemia, nausea and fatigue (National Cancer Institute). These side effects can be managed and often ease after treatment is completed.

What are the odds?

The majority of the medical community will deal with your condition in terms of percentages. Remember when they used to talk about the weather in a very vague way?

There was "a slight chance of rain" or "a good chance it will be a nice day tomorrow" or "a good chance of rain but a severe locust warning." Then one day the forecasters switched over to a percentage for the weather report and that's pretty much what they do now with cancer as well. When I first went to my family doctor and they found a lump, there was a 10% chance of a malignancy. When they did a biopsy it was 20%, and when they did a couple of ultrasounds it went to 45%. Right before surgery it went to 90%. I told this to my naturopath who said to me "Rob if they're saying you've got a 90% chance of having it, then it's actually 100% and they don't want to scare the hell out of you." Fair enough. I appreciated his honesty. Regardless of whether your chances go up or down, you will hear the probability of malignancy expressed in percentages. I began to get concerned when I had more of a chance of malignancy than I had of completing a flush on the river (35% according to Phil Laak, Doyle Brunson, and Daniel Negreanu, all of whom I would like to play with sometime. If, by chance, you guys ever need someone to show up for a game with a $20 buy in, let me know.)

The "C" Word

Another thing I noticed during pre-treatment is that the people giving you care will avoid using the word cancer as often as possible. They will use the word "malignancy" a great deal or the terms "sickness" or "growth" as back-ups, but rarely will they come out with the word cancer. I imagine they've all gone to a conference where some psychiatrist told them that when they talk to patients they need to soften the blow and not throw "The Big C" around too much.

You may hear these euphemisms so much that after a

while it becomes a bit funny. I would occasionally just play a game with the health professionals just to see if I could make them uncomfortable. I'd be talking to a nurse or other health care provider and they might say, "Well, how are you doing with your malignancy?" I'd respond with "You mean how am I doing with my cancer?" They'd look startled and eventually continue. It's a strangely powerful space to be in. Often times they were more uncomfortable with the word than I was. After a while, you will get used to the whole concept of dealing with this disease and you'll almost enjoy watching everyone else dance around it.

"Paging Dr. Murphy....Paging Dr. Murphy..."

I hate to say this but, during this time of tests and diagnosis, there is a very good chance that "they" will lose your files and tests results. You are in fact dealing with a very large bureaucracy and things out of your control will just happen. Paper will get lost, coffee might be spilled on your X-ray results, or a Spaniel with a bladder problem will eat the intern's homework. I have never been a proponent of Murphy's Law but in this one instance it sure seemed like Murphy himself was behind the scenes somewhere pulling the strings. There is very little you can do about this except just realize that it is part of the deal. Eventually, you will get your results back and your doctor will be in town and the receptionist will find your file under her most recent edition of *Weights and Measures Magazine*.

A Fun Example

After I had my biopsy, I had an appointment with an ear nose and throat specialist, who I will call "Doctor Dick", and not because his first name is Richard. Dr. Dick, to whom I had been referred by my family doctor, was supposed to diagnose my condition and inform me of my course of treatment. I had to wait months for this appointment, so I had my notebook with my questions at the ready. When I finally sat in his office, Dr. Dick barely greeted me except to acknowledge my name, then he shuffled through my file and said, "Didn't you get a biopsy? Where are the test results?"

I assured him that I had and that the results should be in my file. He looked in the file again. I very gently suggested that perhaps there had been some miscommunication between the test facility and his office. He looked at me with something like disgust and said, "My people don't make mistakes." He picked up the phone and called out to his receptionist "Do you have Robert's biopsy results?" After a prolonged pause it became clear that they did not have said results. Dr. Dick looked at me as if my Saint Bernard had just crapped on his lawn and said, "The test facility must have screwed up. Did you tell them to send it to this office?"

"Yes, I believe I did."

"Well, it's not here! You'll have to contact the people who did the tests and get them to resend it."

I was pretty shocked by this order but I agreed to hunt down my own biopsy. I looked down at my notebook to ask a question or two while my remarkably sympathetic medical professional was in the room.

"So, doctor, can you tell me how long it would take me to recover from..."

"Look, I can't do a thing for you until I get the results back. This will all just be a waste of time. When you get the biopsy results, call my office and set up an appointment, I'll see you in a month or so."

"I just had some questions," I stammered. Fortunately, I didn't have to find many more words.

"Look, you're my last appointment of the day and as you can see its beautiful out and I've got an early dinner reservation." He motioned to the door for me to leave. I gathered up my notebook and assorted anxieties and left his office. This time, I am actually not exaggerating this conversation. This "specialist" seemed to have remarkably little concern for his patients and as a bonus had all the bedside manner of Genghis Kahn.

Eventually I tracked down the results and arranged to have them resent to the impressive Dr. Dick. It was quite surprising to me that I had to do this legwork myself, but it seemed easier than complaining about it. In the meantime however, I went back to my family doctor who had referred me to the specialist in the first place.

I consider my family doctor a friend, so I couldn't help but wonder why he gave me a referral to a doctor with the people skills of a rabid badger(Genghis Kahn? Rabid Badger? My editor wanted me to pick one, but I like both). I mustered up my courage and went to see my excellent family doctor. We'll call him "Dr. F."

Dr. F explains the Bureaucracy
A very busy medical professional named Doctor F walks into exam room #3. Rob sits on the table.

Dr. F:
Hey Rob, What can I do for you?

Rob:
Dr. Dick is an asshole!

Dr. F:
What?

Rob:
He treated me like crap! I know you're a really good

doctor and all, but why would you send me to him. He sucks!

Dr. F:
I know he's an asshole.

Rob:
(Dumbfounded) Wha?

Dr. F:
I can tell by your monosyllabic response that you are surprised by my agreement on this issue.

Rob:
Ya!

Dr. F:
I know he's an asshole. Everybody knows he's an asshole. That's why I referred you to him.

Rob:
Huh?

Dr. F:
It's like this: I had a pretty good idea that your thyroid was giving you trouble and that you may or may not have cancer. I also wanted to get you to a surgeon as quickly as possible and before you can go to a surgeon, you have to go see a specialist who can refer you to a surgeon. So, I sent you to Dr. Dick, who doesn't have a waiting list because, basically, he's an asshole.

Rob:
So, you sent me to him because he's an asshole so I'd get treatment faster?

Dr. F:
Bingo!

Rob:
Oh. Well, thanks, I guess.

Dr. F:
By the way, lose ten pounds.

As you can gather, this whole set of experiences really brightened my outlook. I bring it up to let you know that although most medical professionals are gifted, empathetic and caring folks, some of them are, well, assholes. Fortunately, the ratio of assholes to generous highly skilled professionals is very high (at least 15:1). If you are lucky, you will encounter only doctors who know how to treat people with skill and kindness, but if not, brace yourself and get ready to rant to a sympathetic ear later.

Just Another Life-Changing Day

You might notice that the people working in the test centers are not weeping in sympathy as you enter and leave the room. Although this whole experience is very big news for you, it is actually a very everyday occurrence to the people running the diagnostic equipment and checking you into the waiting room. In fact, while they're working they might also be wondering when in the afternoon they can slip out for a short triple latte Frappucino. I remember getting a biopsy and thinking that the woman was downright cheery about the whole thing. Didn't she know this was a situation of great impact? Didn't she know she had a window to my mortality in her hands? She was much more interested in knowing whether or not I had finished my holiday shopping. It took me a minute to realize that she was a pro and that not everything could be life or death for her. In fact, after a while her casualness really helped to relax me and keep away the screaming-meemies. So, don't be surprised if people are treating your tests and procedures like it's just another day, because to them, it is.

You're Hired!

This whole journey can take more time than you think, with all the appointments and research and waking up at 3 AM. It can feel like you've just been forcibly conscripted into a another job. For a while, researching your treatment, following up with doctors, and getting tests is going to be what you do. Some other things may have to go by the wayside for a bit but once you're healthy again, you'll be able to get back to doing more of the things you love.

Chapter 6

Prepping for Surgery or Treatment

"In three words I can sum up everything I've learned about life. It goes on."
—Robert Frost

In this chapter:

The basics help a lot
The benefits of laughter
Expect to be stupid
Now is the time to ask

Throughout this process, there are huge stretches of time when you will feel like there is nothing you can do but wait. You may miss feeling in the driver seat of your own experience. Well, at this particular time, called pre-surgery, there is a great deal that you can do to help yourself. I actually really enjoyed getting ready for surgery, because the actions I took gave me feelings of autonomy and independence that were very much in short supply at the time.

Here's what I found very useful...

Back to Basics, Baby...

The first thing to prepare for, if you're having any kind of major surgery, is having your basic needs met. I would suggest you make your apartment or house as comfortable for yourself as you can. You're probably going to be out of commission for a while when you come back home and it will do you a world of good if your place is in good shape. You might want to treat preparation for surgery in the same way that you get ready for a trip (granted, this would be a very lousy trip, where you get stuffed full of bad drugs and then run over by a truck, but still, a trip is a trip.)

You might feel fine now, but when you get out of the hospital, you will feel like you spent the weekend wrestling drunken syphilitic bears, so at the very least you might want to stockpile your favourite foods. Freeze your favourite meals or casseroles. Immediately after surgery, comfort foods reign supreme. I go crazy for cooked chocolate pudding, not the kind that you get out of the package, but the kind where you have to boil the milk first and then after you cook it, the skin forms on top and you skim the top layer off while the pudding cools and the dark gooey goodness hits your belly while it's still warm. (Excuse me, I think I need a moment.) This, to me, is chocolate-flavoured morphine. I had a bunch of this ready to go post surgery and was I ever glad I had stocked up. Whatever the equivalent of cooked chocolate pudding is for you, get a bunch of that. I know, I know, it's fattening and you'll gain weight but really, you just had cancer surgery. You've got the rest of your life to run on a damn treadmill.

Oh Yeah, Health

Having just done a commercial for chocolate pudding,

it's probably time to balance that out with something your doctor would agree with. Get yourself a bunch of healthy food as well and things that are easy to prepare. You might want to plan for a good solid week of meals without having to go to the store. If you are lucky enough to have someone going through this with you, then they can pick stuff up that you didn't think of beforehand. If there's something that you've forgotten, call up someone on your list who can get it for you.

Also, do your laundry. Have virtually all the clothes in your house clean because you're not even going to be able to think about it for a while and being able to put on clean socks on Day 7 will really help you.

It will be really useful to take care of as much practical life stuff before hand as you can. Make sure you have your rent, mortgage and the hydro bill either taken care of or in the hands of someone who will take care of it. Intelligent thought and the ability to manage your own affairs will come back to you, but it's going to take a while. Two weeks should be a good amount of time for you to get the cobwebs out of your head after your procedure and give you enough time to get your faculties back so you can look after your own affairs again.

Have some cash on hand. A couple hundred bucks stashed away for post-surgery needs will make life a lot easier. If you get to the point where you need to go outside and get something, it will do you a world of good to be able to skip the trip to the bank machine and go straight to the store. You also might want to get some food delivered or take a cab to a loved one's place, so a bit of cash will be very handy. Even if you don't use it, it's good just knowing its there.

Make Me Laugh, Dammit!

"The art of medicine consists of keeping the patient amused while nature heals the disease."
—Voltaire

We've been told it for years and medical science backs it up: laughter heals. In an article entitled "Humor and Health" by Paul E. McGhee, PhD, he states:

"It's clear that there is something about humor and laughter that causes the immune system to "turn on" metabolically and do more effectively what it is designed to do—promote health and wellness in the face of internal or external threats."

McGhee also goes on to explain how laughter can boost different aspects of the immune system, reduce stress and can be used effectively in pain management.

Cancer Treatment Centers of America offer "Laughter Therapy" to their patients as part of a course of treatment, and furthermore, according to McGhee, *"over a dozen studies have now documented that humor does have the power to reduce pain in many patients."*

With so much medical science backing up the fact that laughter heals, we should take advantage of it through every stage of this journey. A very useful strategy is to get a bunch of funny DVDs that you really enjoy. Get some comedies, or just your favourite feel good movies, and sock them away so you can pull them out on the second or third day that you're home. They will make a world of difference.

Here are some suggestions...

Funny Stuff
1: Anchorman
2: Bill and Ted's excellent Adventure

67

3: Dodgeball
4: Monty Python and the Holy Grail
5: Any of Eddie Izzard's stand-up videos.

Another resource for some great comedies is the Film Institute List of 100 best American comedies, or search "100 years 100 laughs" on Google.

If a movie is a bit too much of a commitment for you, you can always head to youtube (www.youtube.com) and type in the name of virtually any stand up comedian to get a look at some great bits. Chris Rock, Eddie Izzard, Dane Cook and many others have clips posted that you can watch anytime, night or day.

Believe it or not, video games—that's right, video games—can be really useful as an effective pain management strategy. A study that was done at Wheeling Jesuit University showed that kids who played video games actually dealt with pain far better than children who did not: "*This study found that playing video games significantly distracts people from painful stimulation. This could be a great adjunct to pain management in children.*" (That sound you hear right now is an executive at Microsoft running straight to the marketing department.)

A good fantasy can work wonders as well. I ended up watching the entire *Lord of the Rings* Trilogy over a few nights when I was in pretty rough shape. Every night I'd watch those hobbits fight those orcs and wonder why the elves got all the hot chicks—and I'd feel much better afterwards.

Whatever your distraction is, be it comedies or video games, use it. Indulge in it. You deserve it and contrary to what we were told growing up, playing a video game and laughing at fart jokes can actually be good for you.

Packing for the Hospital

It's pretty simple to pack for this journey; you might want to bring a light novel with you or maybe a favourite magazine. If they give you general anesthetic and you're on morphine or some other opium-based pain killer, you're really not going to be up for *Harpers*. If you are, my hat is off to you, but I found it best to go for the easiest stuff I could find. Bring your MP3 player because having your own music will give you some kind of autonomy and can really comfort you during your hospital experience.

Expect to Be Stupid

Post-surgery, you will have anesthetic floating around in your body that can alter virtually every experience you have. These drugs are strong enough to knock you out while a surgical team does a mambo in your thorax so they've got to be pretty powerful. Given that, and the fact that it puts you under in about five seconds, you've got a pretty good indication that the anesthetic will hang around in your system for a while.

Thanks in Advance

OK. If you really want to be a superstar for your caregiver, here's something you can do for them *before* you go in to surgery. If you are up to it you can write them a letter thanking them for all their help in advance. It could go something like this...

Hey Spouse, Friend, Brother, Sister,

I'm probably completely unconscious now and you've

been looking after me for about a week but I just wanted to thank you for all the remarkable things you've done in the last while. I know there have probably been times when you have been at the end of your rope and wondered how you were going to go on, but you did and I thank you for that. I'm probably quite grumpy and incoherent right now. In fact, I might be quite challenging to be around, but it really helps me that you are here. Many thanks.

Love, George.

(You might want to omit this last bit if your name is not, in fact, George. Otherwise, it's going to confuse everyone.)

When you are well enough, insist that your caregiver go out and do something for him or herself. Suggest that they go to a movie or take out a friend or go out to dinner. If you're not well enough to be on your own, get someone to come over and be with you while they go out. They need it. They have been through the wringer watching you go through the wringer, and they need some space from the whole thing. They've been on overdrive for a long time looking after you and they need a break from the hospitals, the doctors and even you. Very likely, your caregiver will insist that they're OK and that they are fine being with you 24/7. Gently insist that they go out for a bit. Tell them that you will be fine for a couple of hours with the skin on your pudding and your well-worn copy of *Anchorman*. You could even take some of that loose cash on hand and say "Hey go and buy yourself a meal or a coffee." If the person looking after you is your lover, the relationship has probably been unbalanced for a while, but no matter how wonderful they've been, they still have needs. A bit of time away from the whole situation, even if it's just a couple of hours, will do them a ton of good.

Have a Contact List

Have a list of your loved ones' names and contact numbers prepared before you go for surgery and post it somewhere very handy, like your fridge. You may have to ask for help to do some simple but important things. Having a friend come in to take care of laundry, do some cleaning and cook you a good meal can be very useful. Funnily enough, the people in our lives usually are glad to do this kind of thing for us. Many times the tricky part is not getting them to do it, but actually asking them.

I really needed my laundry done about ten days after surgery but I was too weak to get the job done. At the time, I lived on the third floor of a low rise and the laundry was in the basement. I just didn't have the strength to go up and down the stairs a few times to get my clothes clean. It was too embarrassing to have my brother drive into town and carry my laundry for me. He would have done it in a heartbeat (he's that kind of guy) but I didn't know how to ask for help. You might have to swallow your pride for a while and ask for assistance on some pretty basic things. The ability to ask for help will be a great skill to develop, because chances are you're going to need it. Don't worry; people will be glad to do virtually anything for you. You just have to ask them.

How to Ask

Alright, this might seem remarkably goofy but we're going to give an example of how to do this. Why? Because clearly, our society worships independence and strength. As a result of this, when we are in a position when we actually need to ask for help, it can be difficult for us to do so. Kicking cancer's ass takes a support system and setting this up in advance can make it a lot easier. You might start like this...

"Hey how are you?"

"I'm good."

"OK, You've heard I'm going in for cancer treatment?"

"Of course, I'm so sorry…"

"Thanks! After surgery, I'm going to be in recovery for a bit and I'm really going to need a hand because I may not be able to look after myself for a while, so could you do some things for me?"

"Oh God, of course."

"Thanks a ton, I hate to ask, but I might need help with laundry and shopping. Could you help me with that?"

"Of course. I'd be glad to."

"Thanks a lot. Could you give me a call a week after surgery?"

"Sure."

"Oh, and when you come by, could you bring the Jell-o mould that you borrowed last fall?"

"Of course."

There, you see? That wasn't that bad at all. I know it seems a bit funny, but setting this stuff up before hand can really help out. Most folks really *want* to do something for you but really don't know what to do. When people say "I really wish there was something I could do to help," they usually mean it. You might want to say something in response like "Well, as a matter of fact there is…"

A few things they might be able to help you with are giving you a hand with laundry, shopping for food, cleaning your place up a bit, driving you to a follow-up appointment, hanging out with you for an evening, watching a dumb movie with you and going to lunch when you are up for it. I'm not advocating that you take advantage of people, far from it. I am assuming that you are a generous person who would pretty much do anything for a friend in the same situation. Well, your friends and family want to do the same for you, so give them that opportunity.

The good news about prepping for surgery is that it is fundamentally proactive and gives you power. In addition, getting yourself properly prepared really helps your recovery in the long run.

Chapter 7

My Hospital Experience

"I learned a long time ago that minor surgery is when they do the operation on someone else, not you."
—**Bill Walton**

In this chapter:

My hospital experience
Gosh, I'm a patient!
Did you hear the one about the nurse from Transylvania?
If you can, go private

This is the story of my hospital experience. Everyone's will be different, of course, but I'm hoping some of this is universal in nature and may be useful to you in preparing for your treatment.

I remember how it was when I went in. I was completely prepped and ready to go, my parents had come down from London (a three hour drive) and my girlfriend at the time was there as well. I was feeling pretty cheery about the whole thing, actually. I was determined to make it as much an adventure as possible. I went through the bureaucratic process of being admitted to the hospital and was taken to my room which had three other guys in it. They were all much older than myself and (so I thought) much sicker than I was. One poor guy had had a hip replacement and was moaning in pain, another guy was recovering from abdominal surgery, and the gentleman across from me had been there for twenty days or some ridiculous amount of time like that. It struck me that I was entering the hospital while still being essentially very healthy. With my particular kind of malignancy (thyroid) there were no real overt symptoms. I wasn't limping or anything like that. You wouldn't look at me and say "Oh look at that guy, he's got cancer."

I went into my room and they gave me the standard bare-assed hospital gown and told me to get into it. I remember looking around my ward at the other sick guys and thinking "Damn, at least I'm not as bad as that. This will be a piece of cake." I sat and waited for surgery until the suspense was almost too much and right then the orderly came to get me. Now, I believe in some great force in the universe that says "Hello" to us by throwing a bit of synchronicity our way. The orderly came in and wheeled the gurney in front of me. At that point, I knew that the hospital trip had really begun and there was no going back. I jumped onto the gurney and asked his name.

"Moses," he replied.

"What?"

"Moses."

I started to laugh my ass off.

"Moses, I would follow you anywhere!"

He broke into a huge grin and pushed me through the hallway. It seems I was off on a trip through the desert.

The Patience of a Patient

Now it's a funny thing about the hospital: once I had the gown on and the I.D. bracelet on my wrist, there was no doubt that I was a PATIENT. I was no longer a self sufficient, independent guy who could ride his bike through downtown traffic and give the couriers a run for their money. No, I was a patient; someone to be pulled, prodded and pushed into the proper room and given Jell-o at specific times. I realized this as I was in the elevator lying on the gurney surrounded by people going to different floors.

I nervously tried to make conversation about the weather with somebody who was not a patient and they just looked at me like I was some kind of freak. I definitely got the message. They were uncomfortable talking with someone who was in the blue gown.

I was wheeled into yet another waiting area that was essentially the warm up circle for the operating room. My girlfriend at the time stayed with me and held my hand because I was a bit scared.

Finally they came to get me. I asked the nurse if I could walk into the operating room myself and apparently that was OK. So I got up and walked into a surprisingly large bright room filled with people in masks. I was introduced to everyone and made some quip like "Hi, my name is Rob and I'll be your patient today." Someone laughed and I was very glad they did. I got up on the table and was surrounded by five or six people.

Everyone was very good to me. They were very conscious that I was scared even though I was joking around (or maybe even *because* I was joking around), so they used my first name a lot and explained every step as we prepared for the operation. I was hooked up to a heart monitor and heard it ping away as I waited for surgery to begin. They put the mask over my face and got me to count backwards from a hundred (which is really a joke—they should just say "Now you're going to be unconscious and there's nothing you can do about it." I got to 98 and that was it).

The next thing I knew, I was staring at a clock that was telling me that six hours had passed. I felt incredibly groggy and I was surprisingly pissed off. The first thing I did was try to get up. Don't do this. It's not advisable at all and will bring nurses scrambling to you in very short order. A voice came over the intercom that informed the visitors to the hospital that in fifteen minutes it would be time to go. At that point I had not seen my folks yet and I was really worried that they would be kicked out before I had a chance to tell them that I was alright.

In my groggy state, I thought my parents would probably leave the hospital because they wouldn't want to disturb the other patients. Of course at this point I thought my best option was to try to get up out of bed. *Semiconscious after major surgery? Completely stoned on pain medication? In a foggy rage? Time for a stroll!* Fortunately, someone was there to make sure that I wasn't going to go very far. I have no idea who she was and I never saw her again but she stood there and assured me that my family would not be kicked out and that I would see them after I went upstairs to my room. I then started talking (in a very hoarse voice) about how I was so pissed that I had cancer, and what did I do to deserve this, and about how unfair all of it was. I wasn't very coherent at the time so I'm pretty sure that a lot of it was gobbledygook but it meant so much to me that this person listened so attentively while I prattled on.

Hello Morphine!

I was the last one in the huge surgery recovery room and finally I was wheeled up to my room. My family was there and we had a short visit. My return to my room was much different than my arrival that morning. I was very definitely a patient now and quite incapable of taking care of myself. My family stayed for a while and then left me alone for the night. Now I had the pleasure of being on morphine for the next couple of days, and I have to say that this particular poppy-based drug is remarkable. Through the night there was constant noise that would normally make sleep impossible. The poor old bastard next to me was in constant pain and couldn't stop moaning. Machines beeped, monitors monitored and we all tried to get a few hours of rest while the nurses came in periodically to attend to us. Because of the beautiful morphine, I wasn't so bothered by all of this. I was aware of all the activity when I was awake, but it felt a lot like I was floating down a beautiful warm river. And when I actually was able to sleep, my dreams were these vivid, electric, ten-second conversations with characters that would form in front of me briefly, say a few words and then dissipate to be replaced by someone else. They'd say something like, "The instant pudding is next to the Prime Minister" and then they'd be gone. Even though I was drugged, I still had some pain that peaked at about 4 AM. I wasn't conscious enough to complain about it, but I certainly felt it and here's where another one of the great differences between medical professionals comes in...

Ah Yes, Morning...

I woke up and met my nurse in the morning, I forget her name now and that's just as well. She told me that she was from the part of the Ukraine commonly known as

Transylvania. *The* Transylvania. The next thing she said to me was, "Oh Rob, I am so proud of you! I only gave you one milligram of morphine last night instead of the two milligrams that I could have given you. I knew that you could do it!"

This nurse was very professional and gave me very good care, however, when I've just had major surgery and my body feels like it has been run over by a Mack truck, I want as many drugs pumped into my system as is legal in my current jurisdiction. She went off duty shortly and a nurse came on who was thrilled to give me all the drugs I could stand.

There really is no need to be a tough guy through this at all. If you're in pain, ask for some help. You're not being a bother, your body has just experienced a pretty heavy trauma and it needs some help to get through the next while.

Sometime after my liquid breakfast, I was lying in my bed looking like two hundred pounds of traumatized crap. The gentleman across from me, who I'd thought looked so rough the day before, made a great effort to lift up his arm in a silent wave to me. He even smiled a bit. It was the simplest and most profound gesture I've yet seen. Suddenly, I was one of them. We were all in this together and had our own pain whether it was cancer, a replaced hip, or abdominal surgery. We were all just the guys in the room trying to make it through the day, hour by hour.

An Excursion to the Bathroom

That morning was a little weird. I had been told that I would be asked to go to the bathroom and that I needed to urinate. A buddy of mine had told me before my trip to the hospital that if I wasn't able to pee that they would fit me with a catheter. Youch! This was not an experience that I was looking forward to, so I made it my mission to fulfill this requirement as soon as possible. Funny, it had never been a major project for me to urinate before, but it certainly was now. I sat on that toilet for a good fifteen minutes and prayed for any liquid at all to come out of me. I know it's not a pretty image, but in the end, I was able to get everything working alright.

Yes this was a bit rough, but I got through it and if I did it, so can you. Also there are many different kinds of surgery and everyone reacts differently to these treatments. My particular surgery was a complete thryroidectomy but some surgeries are more invasive, and fortunately, some are less so. If you're prepared and know what to expect, you're a lot better off.

To Semi-Private or Not to Semi-Private

Because of my health care benefits, I was given the option of getting a semi-private room. It hadn't been available the first night, but I was moved into it near the end of my first day after surgery. As luck would have it, I was the only one in the room so actually, I had a private room for my second night. Now, as much as I really liked the guys in the old room and I felt a profound sense of brotherhood with them, going from a ward room to a semi-private (but technically private) room was like walking from a shack into a suite at the Four Seasons. It was actually possible for me to rest. The only heart monitor was the one hooked up to my ticker, and if anyone was moaning, it was me. The Transylvanian Lieutenant was nowhere to be found and I had a nurse who actually gave me extra drugs on occasion. Hallelujah. The upshot of all of this is if you can get yourself a semi-private room, go for it, even if you have to pay for it yourself. I think the difference to me would have been $190 out of my own pocket had I not been insured, and I would have gladly paid that given the difference in experience. These were the circumstances in the Canadian healthcare system; it may be different where you are.

Check Out, Nine Items or Less

Checking out of the hospital can be a bit of a dance with the health care bureaucracy. They will offer you a wheelchair when you are in the process of leaving. My advice is to sit in it as long as you can. You're probably thinking "I've been in the hospital now for two days (or whatever it happens to be) and I feel fine! I don't want the damn wheelchair!" Oh but you will. That crazy old anesthetic is still coursing through your body and you will be tired before you know it.

The process of checking out will entail more waiting around than you think, and after that, you may have a trip to the pharmacy to get your new prescriptions. All of this coupled with the fact that your stamina will be remarkably lower than you are used to necessitates the use of that damn wheel chair for as long as possible. So be patient. You'll be home soon. And the next stage of your recovery can begin.

Chapter 8

Recovery: When You First Get Home

"When the Japanese mend broken objects, they aggrandize the damage by filling the cracks with gold. They believe that when something's suffered damage and has a history it becomes more beautiful."
—**Barbara Bloom**

In this chapter:

Cut yourself a lot of slack
How long is this gonna take?
The first shower
My adventures without medication
Have more than one source of information

Cut Yourself a Lot of Slack

Surgery itself doesn't last that long. In fact, to you it will probably seem like it happens in an instant. My brother asked me if I had any awareness at all during my surgery. I explained that I was cognizant of nothing, and there was only blackness during the whole procedure. I counted backwards from 100 as per my anesthesiologist's instructions but only got to 98 and then woke up feeling like Jim Morrison on New Year's Day. (Except that instead of just drinking too much, Jim had apparently wandered off the night before and questioned the sexuality of the leader of the Hell's Angels.) For others with less invasive surgery, it can be a lot easier.

Surgery is a relatively brief event that everyone is concerned about, and rightly so, but the period called *post-surgery* is what separates the wimps from the tough guys. Friends and family are very worried about your well-being leading up to and right after the big event; however, the long road back to health during post-surgery is what takes the most courage, patience and strength. Again, our familiar mantra of "one day at a time" is the way to go. Recovery begins the second you wake up after your operation and every small step you take after that will get you closer to being healthy again.

How Long is This Gonna Take?

I found it very strange that there were so many different estimates on recovery time. My surgeon told me it would be about a month until I felt alright again. My GP told me I would be off work for about two weeks and then I would be fully productive again with no problems at all. I was told frequently that this was an "easy" cancer and that I would feel exactly like I did before the surgery in seven days. (By the way, it's inadvisable to tell someone they have an "easy" cancer. It's kind of insulting.)

People around the proverbial water cooler will tell you that Uncle Marvin had the same thing a year ago and he was back to hog calling in under three days. But you're not Uncle Marvin and you hate hog calling so your recovery time may be different. You just never know how your body is going to react, so if it takes a bit longer than you think, cut yourself some slack. What's more important than completely recovering from this thing so you can get on with your life?

When you get home, you will feel much better just because you're in your own space again. If you live with someone, they may be able to give you a hand over the next while, be they a spouse, family member or roommate. If you live alone, you might ask a friend to sack out on the couch for a few days just to be there with you. Failing that, have someone that you can call night or day if you are scared, lonely or even a bit confused. The first few days at home you will probably sleep like crazy. Chances are you will still be full of anesthetic and your body will have suffered a pretty big trauma so you will probably spend a lot of time completely unconscious.

The First Shower

One of the most enjoyable experiences you will have once you are out of the hospital is your first shower back home. You will love it. It feels so unbelievably good to get that hospital stink washed off of you that you will probably stand in the steamy water for an alarming amount of time until your caregiver knocks on the door and asks "Are you OK?" Through the sauna-like conditions, you will mumble that you are in fact having the best damn shower of your life. You'll probably climb into bed and sleep for a good solid six hours or so because standing up in that shower is probably the most energy you have exerted in a long while.

Getting Things Moving

Ah yes, constipation.

There really is no delicate way to put this, but if you've been prescribed morphine or some other pain-killing opiate then in all likelihood you will be constipated. This is because opiates tend to radically impede your digestive system and also because your body has been completely slowed down by the anesthetic. After a few days of this "congestion on the highway of life", you will probably need some kind of laxative to get things moving again. I found that suppositories worked very well for me. Some folks find suppositories to be too strong, so you might want to find a gentler laxative. Once your body begins cleaning itself out again, you will begin to feel much better, and we won't have to have this conversation again.

Hungry?
In terms of food right after surgery, go for stuff that is really simple. Yogurt, scrambled eggs and that pudding you have stored away is great. If you're not ready to eat yet don't worry about it, but if you do, go for things that are easy to prepare and digest.

Beep! You have 43 new messages.
Friends and family may have left a bunch of messages on your machine wishing you well. Don't respond to them yet unless you really want to, because right now everything you do needs to serve you. End of story. You are at a stage of recovery that takes a ton of energy and your body will want to sleep and rest. My rule of thumb is: When in doubt, go to sleep. If you're sitting and watching a rerun of "Star Trek: TNG" and you wonder if maybe you should go to bed for a while, then you should. Chances are you'll be unconscious faster than…zzzzzz.

You will probably stay in this state for a few days, but after a while (for me it was day 3) you will start to feel a little better and want to venture out. Your doctor most likely will have told you to go for walks. Medical professionals are crazy for us to go for walks during recovery. It's a very simple exercise that is very good for your body and will help to move that anesthetic out of your system. You might not *want* to do this. In fact, you might feel less like exercise than any other time in your life; however you really should get yourself out of your house or apartment and go for a stroll. The speed at which the world is moving will blow your mind. You will be walking very slowly and old Mr. Perkins from next door will race by you with the comparative energy of a Tasmanian devil.

Just seeing people in your neighborhood will be a bit of a thrill. A simple hello to the postman might be enough to lift your spirits completely, while a trip to the variety store to get some milk and cookies might seem like a day's work. After a few nods to folks in your neighborhood, you'll probably need to go home and rest like you just ran a marathon. With all the walks, sleeping and the comfort food, you will make progress over time.

Going Off Cytomel: My Adventures without Medication

Occasionally in recovery, we run into a tough time. Here's one of mine. A while after the surgery, I thought I was doing pretty well. I was getting myself back together again and I could feel that I was recovering. In my experience, as part of the post-op treatment for thyroid cancer, they have to put you on a drug to replace what your removed thyroid used to do. This drug regulates the body and makes sure that everything in your body does what it should. So, I was on one of these drugs called Cytomel and seemed to be adapting to it pretty darn well. My doctor told me that I had to go off this drug so for about nine days so that he could see if there were any cancer cells left in my body. The doctor told me that there would be some "slight discomfort" and "grogginess" involved, and that I shouldn't make any big decisions during this nine day period.

I stopped taking the pills like a good patient and went home. I felt pretty good for a few days and was even able to ride my bike while doing errands. Ha! I thought to myself, this isn't so bad. Then I started to feel a bit funny. My digestion slowed down, and I felt just a little bit stupid. I was still able to function but I didn't have my usual edge.

Then a couple of days later, things really started to go downhill. My whole body began to feel much slower. My ability to think abstractly was greatly affected and I started to drop things a lot. I thought this was a bit alarming so I contacted a local thyroid support group on the Web. I was able to talk to a woman who asked me how far I'd gone without taking the drugs. When I told her I was about six days in, she said, "Oh boy are you ever in for something!"

"Really? What?" I replied thickly.

She explained that I would be really messed up for the rest of my time off the drug. She said that it was very common for people to do crazy things like lose their car keys in the freezer. She insisted that I not ride my bike anymore and batten down the hatches. Over the next few days I felt like hell, I got progressively more stupid and slow. My voice even dropped a couple of tones. For entertainment, I watched squirrels play outside my window for hours. I even caught myself staring at the TV screen when it was off.

My Dad and Mom are awesome.

I called my parents at one point in tears and sobbed on the phone for a while to them just because I was scared and confused. They did the right thing, which was to listen and offer support. I suffered through the last day and went to the doctor and he took one look at me and apologized to me for putting me through that. This was all very nice of him to say, but what I really needed to know was how it was *actually* going to be *beforehand*. I needed to know that I'd feel stupid, that I'd really not be able to think much at all and that tying my shoes would be a major challenge. In fact, the worst primetime sitcoms were very entertaining to me at that time and I truly felt like they offered valuable insight into the human condition. Yes, I was that impaired.

Have More Than One Source of Information

I guess what I'm trying to say to you is that sometimes your medical professional won't really give you the whole story. I'm not saying you should always assume the worst, far from it. I am saying that it is very useful to make sure that you educate yourself along the way. A former patient or survivor may have insights and experience that your doctor, who has never had cancer, might not have.

(By the way, I checked out fine on the test and the doctor put me back on the meds again. I remember waking up in the morning and feeling my brain kick in. Abstract thought returned and my love for the average sitcom left, all in the very same hour.)

Chapter 9

Recovery: Further Down the Road

"My doctor gave me six months to live, but when I couldn't pay the bill he gave me six months more."
—**Walter Matthau**

In this chapter:

Celebrate your victories
The Expanding Circle
Why am I stoned at lunch?
What's that feeling below my waist?
Dealing with follow-up appointments

Celebrate Your Victories

As you continue to heal, celebrate even the small victories that you have along the way. You might not feel like you're being very brave, but believe me, what you're doing now is completely heroic. All those people out there who are climbing Kilimanjaro, swimming with great white sharks or wrestling barracudas in order to test their mettle have nothing on you. Coming back from a life-altering experience that is threatening and affecting on so many levels is tougher than climbing any mountain. During this process, you have probably been challenged on physical, emotional, and spiritual levels that the barracuda wrestlers only wish they could deal with. When you come to a new milestone in your recovery (like walking for fifteen minutes without stopping or going to the grocery store by yourself), make sure that you take note and recognize what you've done.

In fact, before bed, I found it really useful to think of two things that went well that day. You might ask yourself "What did I do today to help myself recover?" The answer might be as simple as "I had a two hour nap in the afternoon that felt terrific." or "I went for a walk and smiled at the lady outside the laundromat" and that's fine. In fact, it's excellent. Please keep in mind that this is not a sprint. It's a marathon and marathons take patience. If you're a hard-driving personality who gets a lot done in a day, it's tempting to push too hard and really be ambitious in your recovery. Paradoxically, you'll find you recover quicker if you slow down and make naps a priority. In fact, a nap is one of the most ambitious things you can do for yourself while you get back to health.

Right after treatment your world might be remarkably small. You'll be dopey, semi- conscious and probably quite inactive physically. Initially, you'll find that your bed will be base camp and a trip to the bathroom and back might seem like a two day trek across the Sahara. However, as you get better, your world will expand. After a few days you'll venture out to the couch more. After that, with your daily walks, the circle of your world will expand to your immediate neighborhood and might even include going out to a friend's place. As you get more capable and healthier, you will naturally go out into the world a lot more. Eventually, if things go well, you'll find that your circle re-expands to where it was before you had this challenge in your life.

Exercise? Are You Nuts?

"If we are facing in the right direction, all we have to do is keep on walking."
—**Buddhist Saying**

You should exercise more as you feel you have the ability. Again, don't do an hour on the treadmill the first day (heck, I've *never* done an hour on a treadmill) but as you feel yourself able to do so, up your level of exercise, make the walks a bit longer and maybe stretch your level of stamina a bit more. Do this gently, but do it. Why? First and foremost, exercise acts as a natural antidepressant because it releases serotonin into your brain that will elevate your mood. In fact, exercise is a better antidepressant than any pill on the market. James A. Blumenthal, PhD, made the following conclusions after a study done in 1999: "Our findings suggest that a modest exercise program is an effective, robust treatment for patients with major depression who are positively inclined to participate in it."

Why Am I Stoned at Lunch?

"Consciousness: that annoying time between naps."
—**Anonymous**

About a month into my recovery, I was having lunch with a very good friend of mine at one of our haunts, which is known for really good Mexican food. Chris and I were deciding whether we wanted chicken covered in cheese or beef covered in cheese when all of a sudden a wave of tiredness just rolled right over me. I couldn't even continue ordering my chicken enchilada and I had to ask the waitress to come back in a minute or two. In fact, I didn't just feel tired, I felt stoned. It was as if Bob Marley was playing a concert in my head while Peter Tosh was warming up backstage in the rest of my body. I managed to get through lunch speaking in monosyllabic bursts of dialogue until my buddy dumped me in a cab and sent me home to sleep. It was only later that I realized that a fat cell or two must have metabolized and that the residual anesthetic that had been stored inside the cell or cells had been released into my system. There was nothing for me to do but go home and sleep it off. You might find this happens for you as well. One minute you feel fine and the next you feel like you're asleep on your feet.

Not Many Doctors Know About This...

At the time of writing, this sleepy phenomenon is not widely talked about in the medical community. I was very fortunate that a family friend of mine named Dr. Margot Roach who teaches internal medicine spoke with me about a month after my surgery. She explained that it was very common for people to feel very tired and groggy up to six months after an operation involving general anesthetic because these drugs are still active in your system. I was tired for months after surgery and thought that there was something really wrong with me. It was very relieving to find that this fatigue was the result of my body *still* reacting to the drugs.

A strategy to help you get through this faster is to drink a lot of water as it will help flush you out and get a lot of the residual medication out of your system. A good rule of thumb is to drink an ounce of water for every pound of body weight that you have. I'm about 180 pounds (OK OK, 200...) so I drink about 180 ounces of water a day or about 3 liters of water every twenty four hours. I know that seems like enough water to sink the Bismarck but once you drink this amount you'll find that your body will adapt to it and you won't be going to the bathroom every fifteen minutes.

All of this fluid helps to flush the toxins from your system that have built up through the course of your illness.

Exercise will also help your body cleanse the drugs from your cells. Getting rid of the residual anesthetic takes a while and will require patience. Right when you think you're going to feel tired forever, your body will finally flush it out and you'll feel OK again.

Hey Friend!

Now that you're feeling a little better, you'll probably want to be a bit more social but if you go to a huge Halloween party with all of your rambunctious buddies dressed as superheroes you might be completely overwhelmed. Everybody in a party situation will be so happy to see you after your illness that you will get tons of hugs and a bucket of attention. You probably don't need or want a crowd of people hanging around, asking a gazillion questions and slapping you on the back, so start slowly with the socializing as well. One option is to go out to lunch with a family member or friend. This is a much easier situation to control than a large social occasion because at any point with a friend or family member you can say, "Hey great seeing you, but I'm a bit more tired than I thought and I need to hit the road." They will understand, of course; that's why you're close to them. After you do well at this, you can see a couple of friends at a time and *then* maybe you can handle a more demanding social situation like going to church or seeing some folks at a party. When you do go out socially, always do so with the understanding that you can leave at any time without much of an explanation. When you connect with a lot of family or friends at the same time, you might get so much attention and so many good wishes that you'll feel excited, turned on and remarkably loved, which is terrific. When you do go home you'll probably sleep for hours. Your social stamina will be low for a while but, like most things, it will come back over time.

Magic Foot Bath

During my recovery period, it was recommended to me that I take advantage of something called an "Ionic Cellular Cleanse." The benefits, as were explained to me by my naturopath, were that this process would detoxify my body at a cellular level. It goes like this: you place your feet in warm water and an array (which looks like a wand with a cord on the end) is placed in the water with you. The wand then sets up an ionic field within the water and draws out toxins and cellular waste through your feet. The pores in the skin of your feet are the largest in the body and the warm water helps to open them up, allowing more waste material to pass through them, into the water and out of your body. The water can change colour quite dramatically as the toxins leave your body over the course of a 20 minute treatment.

It was suggested I do this after surgery, as there were so many drugs pumped into me during my hospital stay, and my naturopath suggested that these substances may not have been cleansed from my system entirely. My personal results with a cellular cleanse were quite something. After a treatment I usually have a really good three hour sleep, my whole body feels remarkably relaxed and, as a bonus, I have a reduction in joint pain. I recommend this highly to anyone, regardless of whether they've had surgery or not. Some benefits people have reported are:

Reduction in joint pain

Boost to the immune system
Reduction in allergy symptoms
Reduced migraine pain
Reduced arthritic pain
Improved sleep

I used the EB Cellular Cleanse for my treatments. The units themselves are quite expensive, but some chiropractic and naturopathic clinics offer treatments for between $40-60 at a time. If you are interested, just search "EB cellular cleanse therapy" and your city name and hopefully you'll find someone in your area who offers treatments. (And no, I'm not getting any money for recommending this to you. I just think it's remarkably useful.)

What's that feeling below my waist? Oh yeah...

"Sex is not the answer. Sex is the question. 'Yes' is the answer."
—**Swami X**

When you are comfortable with it, it will be time to get back to your sex life again. If you have a sexual partner they are probably hanging around tapping their foot saying, "Ok any time now! Could you rub this?" Physical intimacy is such a beautiful, life- affirming thing that when it pops up in your life again (pun intended) you should dive back in when you feel good about it. Renewed sexual interest is actually a very good sign that things are getting back to normal because it's an indication that your body and spirit have a bit of life energy to spare. If you're getting randy again (or Harry or George), then your system cares about more than just healing itself, so you must really be recovering significantly. Now, you might not be a crazy powerhouse of love initially, so be very gentle with yourself and your expectations. If you are able to actually make love, that's brilliant. If intimacy just involves some touching, holding and caressing, that is amazing too. In fact, even holding someone you love is a remarkably healthy thing to do. There have been a gazillion studies done on the healing power of touch and all of them note that affection is very healthy and will speed your recovery.

If your significant other has been looking after you during this time, they are probably in need of some McLovin as well. They've put their needs on hold for a long time, so gentle physical intimacy is a great way for the two of you to begin giving to each other in a more equal way. Even holding them for a while and telling them that you appreciate them will do a world of good.

Captain Survivor

You now have a new label and category for your resume. Once you are officially out of the woods, you are a "Cancer Survivor." To me this is tantamount to being able to call yourself a Green Beret or a Fire Fighter or even a Fire Fighting Green Beret. You have gone through something that other people are terrified of and lived to tell about it. Some people love this while others would rather forget it, but I wear this moniker very proudly because it makes me feel like I'm in some terrific club filled with death-defying bad-asses. This label also gives you permission to do some things for yourself. Want that bit of expensive chocolate? You deserve it because you're a cancer survivor. Want to ask out that really attractive person who used to intimidate you? Go for it. You deserve to give it a shot because you're a cancer survivor. This label can give you a free pass to all sorts of fun things you want to do in your life, both big and small.

This is a new part of your identity that you need to adjust to, so make it as fun for yourself as possible. After all, you just kicked cancer's ass! You deserve it.

Plan Some Fun

Hope is a tremendous thing. It helps us get through some of the worst times in our lives and is the magic ingredient that moves us forward when things are toughest. One way to nurture hope is to give ourselves very good reasons to keep going through the healing process. As you get better, it will be very useful to give yourself events to look forward to that will keep you rolling along. This might be something as simple as having a goal of attending a party with a bunch of friends, spending the weekend with family, or going to dinner with someone you haven't seen in a very long time. You could arrange to buy yourself an "I Beat Cancer" gift when you get to a certain point in your healing. Once you make the commitment to yourself make sure that you honour it.

When I got healthy, I got myself a new guitar amp with a bunch of very cool sounds, but some other ideas are a painting, a new TV, or even a book you really want. Other options are to have dinner at a really nice restaurant. You also might want to begin to learn some kind of skill like dancing, water-colour painting or small stakes poker.

Roamin' Holiday?

You should go on a holiday!

I know you haven't been able to work for a while and the timing may seem a little funny but it is a great time to get the heck out of "Dodge" for a while. You have been at home a LOT and everything about your existence has been about getting yourself healthy again, so this is a terrific time to reward yourself for getting through what has probably been one of the most difficult times of your life. This could be a huge holiday or one that is much more modest depending on what you feel you can handle both financially and physically. Probably your vacation should really be on the quieter side, like a weekend at a resort or spa rather than a shooter drinking contest in Vegas. Even a couple of days in Niagara Falls at a cottage or whatever place is within driving distance can really recharge your batteries. If you are well moneyed (and more power to you!) you might want to go on a relaxing cruise where most things are taken care of for you. However, if you don't have a lot of cash, you could stay with some friends out of town for a couple of days or even ask a very good friend or family member if you could hang out at their cottage if they're not using it. I know, I know: you could never ask for that but if the situation was reversed and you could help someone by offering a cottage you weren't even using, would you? Of course! So go ahead and ask. Chances are they will be thrilled to say yes. In fact, you can do this in a way that will take the heat off of everyone. Group email or Facebook status update to the rescue! Try this on for size:

Hey Everyone,

I just want to let all of you know that I am doing much better these days and am recovering well. It has been one heck of a journey and I am very thankful for all the help and prayers that I have received. I have a favour to ask that I'm a bit embarrassed about but I'd really like to give it a shot. I could really use a bit of a holiday after all of the time spent recovering from this thing and I wonder if any of you has access to a cottage or second home that is not being used right now. I don't have a lot of money as I haven't been able to work for a month or so, but I would be very grateful for the opportunity to get away from home and clear my head for a while. Thanks very much. I really appreciate it.

Signed,
Me

Not so bad eh? If you saw that note from a friend and you had a place to offer would you want to respond to it? Of course you would! In fact you'd be really happy to have the chance to help out! So, give them the opportunity to do you a good turn.

If you do have some ready cash in your rainy day fund, then by all means use it because there is a price to "free" after all. Get what you need to feel like you have a fresh start and reward yourself for everything you have done and been through.

Follow-Up Appointments

Part of getting better and continuing treatment is going back to the hospital again for follow-up appointments. I found this to be a bit more of a challenge than I thought it would be. In fact, I was surprised to find myself putting off appointments that were crucial to my continued recovery. The doctor would say something like "Hey, make an appointment to see me in a couple of months," and I'd go see him in three or four. I was a bit confused by this at first because I had been very proactive in my healing, so I couldn't figure out why the heck I was avoiding anything to do with medicine. The answer was very obvious and very human: I was scared. Yup. I was frightened of the hospital and the doctors. The prospect of going back in to see my Endocrinologist and sitting there with all the other worried people was very depressing and reminded me of what a hard time I had just gone through. I like to think of myself as a bit of a tough guy but going back to the scene of the crime, to get the "all clear" from my doctor was a bit of a challenge.

Remember all those things you did to help yourself when you were getting tested months ago? Use them. Bring your MP3 player and listen to music you love in the waiting room. Ask a friend along who really cares about you. Make sure you have some time after your appointment to just breathe a while and have a cup of coffee or tea. Remember that all the folks around you in the waiting room are thinking much the same things you are. So, when you go through your follow up appointments breathe deeply, remember that the worst is over and that you are on the road to getting your life back.

You may even find that you feel sad or even cry after your follow up. It's probably just some leftover stress and sadness that you bottled up months ago when you were being very brave. Let it go. You're much safer now and you can release all of that excess baggage. You might be surprised at your depth of feeling at this point, but just let it roll out of you as best you can and be gentle with yourself.

The Goat Path to Health

"Fall seven times, stand up eight."
—**Japanese Proverb**

It's worth stating again that the journey of healing is not like jumping on an interstate and rolling down the highway steadily at 65 mph while you drink a coffee and listen to classic rock. What the heck am I talking about? Well, when you're on a well-groomed highway you can mark your progress in very predictable chunks over regular periods of time. You can look around and say, "Hey, we're going to make it to Cincinnati in two hours and forty five minutes." Healing is not like that. Healing and recovering from cancer is a lot more like being taken away in the middle of the night by a band of roving bandits and dumped in a foreign land by the side of the road where your wallet and keys are stolen. You wake up in the morning, feel hung over and don't really know where you are. When you finally regain coherence, you dust yourself off and use whatever method you can to get back home again. You might ride a donkey at first and then you might have to hitchhike for a while. If you're really lucky, you might grab a train. But progress can be slow at times, fast at others, and seemingly nonexistent on occasion. There will be setbacks and sometimes you'll be completely frustrated with yourself and the whole process. At other times you'll feel your body and spirit coming back to you faster than you thought possible. This irregular progress can be very frustrating, so it's very useful to realize that the unpredictability of your journey is part of the nature of healing.

What's All the Fuss?

You might be out and about now and doing some social things. You will probably find that people will want to fuss over you. Here's how to handle this: let them! Perhaps they will ask you to get together with them for a meal, offer to bring over a casserole, or wonder if they can take you out for a coffee. You should let them do this for a bunch of reasons. You deserve to be treated well by your friends and family.

Also, the folks who are the absolute closest to you might be a bit burned out from looking after you, so if some other people in your life want to contribute, let it happen. They might find it difficult to come right out and say "I really love you, you're really important to me and I'm glad you're alive" so instead of that, they might buy you a Frappucino. Fair enough.

You might also wonder why some friends were not around much while you were sick. Before you un-invite them to your birthday party, you might want to consider the fact that they might have been scared too. Some folks have a very hard time with being around sickness. Thoughts of mortality and seeing people they care about in distress can drive some people around the bend. Often their way to deal with it is to ignore it and pretend it isn't there. This doesn't mean they don't love you, but it might have been the best they could do at the time.

How Did I Get to Be a Hero?

Somewhere along the line someone is going to come up to you and say, "I have no idea how you got through that! You're so brave!" Meanwhile, you've probably been putting one foot in front of the other and trying not to burst into tears when you're in line at the bank. You might not feel very brave. In fact you probably spent a heck of a lot of time being scared, tired, sad and angry, but brave?

This might seem laughable to you, but while you were trying your damnedest to just keep yourself together, other people were watching you and wondering if they could pull it off themselves; as a result you may have a bit of hero status. I'm not saying they're going to close down Main Street and give you a tickertape parade, but some folks will definitely hold you in higher esteem. Some good stuff has to come out of this after all. If you want to tell people about how you got through it, or offer advice on who a good doctor is, go for it. You have now survived an experience that most folks can't touch.

Chapter 10
A Work in Progress

In this chapter:

Get ready for the big question
Changes are a-comin'
Lessons from Joseph (Campbell that is...)
The smaller things really are smaller
What's the big deal about 18 months?

Get Ready for the Big Question

Once you get back on your feet again, people will ask you "How did it change you?" Consider yourself a bit of a rock star at this point, with people asking you the cancer-survivor-equivalent of "How did you write your biggest hit?" And to go from music to mountain climbing, people were probably always asking Sir Edmund Hillary what it was like to climb Mount Everest and how it changed him. You have gone through this incredible process and they want to know what it was like and how they would fare under the same circumstances. They might ask "Do you appreciate every day now? Do you savour everything? Are you a better lover?" I'm still hearing these questions and it's been a couple of years.

The answers are ongoing and keep evolving as my healing process continues. My public response is "Yes, I appreciate every day," and "Yes, I savour everything more than I did before." My private answer is much more layered and complex and chances are yours will be too.

It is very possible that you will change on many levels. For quite a while now (maybe a year or so) you will have been dealing with this. I don't mean that you have been dealing with cancer like you've been dealing with a sore bunion, a poor cable signal or a neighbour whose Shih Tzu keeps crapping on your lawn (maybe that's why it's called a Shih Tzu.) I mean you have been *dealing* with it. I'm talking about a knock-down drag-out experience that has challenged you physically, emotionally, financially and spiritually.

But the funny thing about really impactful emotional experiences is that we really can't help changing if the incidence is big enough. You have probably had to dig very deep to get through this thing called "surviving cancer" And you have gone through so much that some personality shifts may be coming your way.

Your friends and family may come to you after you are feeling a lot better and say "Hey there Buella, I can't help but notice that you're not the same old Buella that you once were." Here's why, you can tell them: "Pre-Cancer Buella" is different from "Post-Cancer Buella". Buella had to kick ass and take down names to get through that experience and now, Buella is looking at things differently and experiencing the world in a unique way, and as a result, this is going to take some adjustment on Buella's part and everybody else's part as well.

But I Don't Want to Change! Do I Have a Choice?

I like to think that we have a lot of freedom in our lives. I can choose what kind of pants I want to wear and what I'm going to have for dessert (cooked chocolate pudding of course) but as to whether or not this experience is going to change me? Frankly, I don't think I had any choice in that at all. It was just too big not to have an effect on my psyche. In your case, you may slightly alter some of your beliefs and perceptions, while some other folks will go through incredible transformative processes where they rework their whole lives. One of our characteristics as human beings is that we grow and change on a regular basis and with all these challenges, this growth may occur at an accelerated pace.

Will I Change in Only One Area of My Life?

Many areas of your life might be altered. I could tell you that all of a sudden you're going to start showing up on time for things, (which wouldn't be bad, but in that case, I'd really rather just buy a damn watch than have cancer) but it's not that simple. Virtually every aspect of your personality will be up for grabs to a certain degree. Everything from having a drink with dinner when you didn't before to deciding whether or not to move to Spain can be affected.

You might find you behave differently financially as well. You might be so turned on by life that you'll go a bit nuts with your money. You might say, "Hey, what the hell, I beat cancer, I can take on anything! And damn it, I deserve a new TV", or a trip to Vietnam, or to have kids, or whatever it is that you have been putting off in your life.

Ladies and Gentlemen, My Good Friend Joseph

I am a fan of a guy called Joseph Campbell. Joseph studied myths and legends from every culture in the world and he found some very strong common threads that ran through a lot of them, which he distilled down into a few basic elements that he called "The Hero Journey." This is explored in detail in a terrific book he wrote called *The Hero with a Thousand Faces*.

The hero journey, as Joseph saw it, goes like this. A young man who is part of a community receives a "call to adventure." The village may be under threat of dragons, or our hero might be on a quest to get a hidden treasure. After he receives "the call to adventure" he goes off, leaves his village and journeys into the unknown. Along the way, in order to slay the dragons or find the treasure, he must go *beyond his former capabilities* in order to win the day.

When our hero defeats the dragons using a magic wand or uses unforeseen strength and cleverness in finding the treasure, he goes *beyond what he thought he was capable of before*. He then returns to his tribe with boons for his community. What is a boon you might ask? A boon is a benefit or something of value. In the above examples it might be the safety of the village, or the treasure. As an added bonus in addition to the boons he brings back, our hero has been *transformed* in the process which is the real point of the hero journey. By going on this challenge, he had to expand himself; he had to dig deep, and go beyond his own expectations in order to triumph over adversity.

How Does This Relate to Me, You Ask?

Well, this hero's journey is not just in stories, folklore

and every Hollywood film you've every seen. It's also echoed and experienced in virtually everybody's life. In fact, I am willing to bet money on the fact that you will go through or are going through your own hero's journey with this health issue right now. I certainly did. It took a long time for me to realize it, but when I did, knowing that I was living through this mythic template made it a lot easier. We'll use my own experience as an example.

I was relatively content in my life before all of this happened. I got the call to adventure in the office of my GP when he was poking around in my neck and said "Hey Rob, what the heck is this lump?" And then I was very definitely off on an adventure that took everything I had to get through. In fact, there were times when I felt completely crazy, lost, scared, sad, infuriated, exhilarated and overwhelmed. Now, you'll remember that, in the hero journey, the main character of the story is transformed in the process. This wasn't his main goal when he set out on this journey. He was going off to fight the dragon or get the treasure. He had no idea that he would transform himself and become more than who he was. That is certainly what happened to me and what may happen for you as well. You will still be who you are and you won't grow a third arm or anything weird like that but, as a result of your journey, you may become a different version of yourself.

The Small Things Are Smaller

One of the great things about being on the other side of this is that, a lot of things will just roll off your back. Maybe you'll be a bit pissed off when you don't get a parking spot or when the pomegranate you just bought seems to be over ripe. But you'll understand that these small things aren't really that bad. You kicked cancer's ass, stared the Reaper straight in the face, and laughed. Who cares about a damn parking ticket? In fact, a while ago I got a traffic ticket on my bike. Yes, that's right, *on my bike*. Sure, I may have run a red light, but still, rules are for cars, not bikes. Funny enough, it didn't make me that mad. You might find that the small things that piss everybody else off won't bother you at all. In fact, you might even be thrilled that you can have the utterly trivial problem of a traffic ticket. I actually thought to myself "What a cool problem to have! I'm on my bike again and healthy enough to break the law." A year before, the only law I could have broken was the one about being incoherent and delirious in a public place. Things were definitely looking up.

Why Is My Moral Compass Spinning?

On the negative side, it might be tricky to make personal choices. Your judgment in this area may be off for a while. You may find that you are doing things that you ordinarily would not do. You might drink more than you used to. You may find that you are louder at parties; you may find you are shy for some reason. I'm not suggesting you take up heroin or get yourself a mohawk but I do think that after you have gone through recovery it is a great time to look at your life and really take stock of how you live it. We make so many decisions everyday just because we are set on autopilot, so this can be a real opportunity to look at how you live your life and make more conscious choices about how you live each day.

A very smart friend of mine once said that sometimes stepping out of your value system is a great way to find out what your values really are. So if you find your values and behaviours are changing a bit, be a bit easy on yourself and forgive yourself as best you can. Once the medical stuff is out of the way, your psyche can't help but readjust as well.

Having just said you might consider a mohawk, I also need to balance this out with a word or two of caution...

I had lunch with a friend who is a survivor and who had a much tougher time than I did with this disease. In fact, her battle with cancer could pretty much be called epic. I related a couple stories to her about how I really wasn't acting like myself and in some cases it seemed like my value system had just gone completely AWOL. She looked at me very calmly and said "that sounds like 18 months to me." She was absolutely right. All of this upheaval in my life had happened about a year and a half after I had been given the all-clear. Apparently it's fairly typical to act a bit erratically at this point in recovery. My advice to you here is BE CAREFUL. I understand that you might be trying out new things, new ways to live and new parts of your personality, but please do your best to continue to treat yourself and those you love well.

Chapter 11
Rebuilding Your Life

"We cannot direct the wind but we can adjust the sails."
—Author Unknown

In this chapter:

Decisions, decisions
What they say about the journey is true
A Word from Mr. T
Yoghurt has it right!
You're soft and strong

Decisions, Decisions

One of the shifts you experience might be that you will be clearer and more focused about your priorities once you get through this thing. I found it much easier to make decisions than I did before. Decisions from what I was going to have for dinner to who I was going to spend a large chunk of my time with became a cinch.

You might find that you are valuing things differently than you did before the sickness. For instance, a year or so after I got over cancer, my nephew Scott and I went on a bike trip from Quebec City to Fredericton, New

Brunswick (this is actually quite far and you should be impressed.) We had planned to go all the way from Quebec City to Halifax, Nova Scotia which would have been about twice as far. We set off on our trip and rode about a hundred kilometers a day and had a blast going on cycling trails through the rugged and beautiful, Canadian landscape. We were flying along, having a great time, when all of a sudden everything went very badly. My gears got messed up, and my bike came to a sudden and very non-glamorous stop. We were unable to continue and ended up hitchhiking.

Now I'm a fairly goal-oriented guy and I must admit that I was pissed at the interruption in our trip as it didn't look like we could continue. However, we stuck out our thumbs, began hitchhiking, and before we knew it, we were both in the back of a pick-up truck with our bikes mashed in beside us while we went a whopping 70 km an hour. We eventually found out my bike couldn't be fixed and ended up loading everything onto a bus to Halifax. I was ridiculously disappointed. Here we were, ready to conquer the world, and then we had to limp into our destination and have my brother Mark pick us up at one in the morning. This was not the triumphant arrival I had expected. However, even though we didn't make our goal of going all the way to Halifax under our own steam, things got really interesting and exciting when everything went wrong. We met some very eclectic and kind people who were thrilled to help us out and got free tours of several east coast car interiors. I'm not saying I'm glad everything went wrong, but there was a point where I did in fact realize that the journey had taken its own turn and that I wasn't in control anymore. The old adage that the journey is the point and not the destination became remarkably clear to me.

In the past I would have thought, "Oh heck it'll be

different next time." Or "We'll do it again and then it will go perfectly." Not anymore. I knew this trip was for keeps, I also knew that the real specifics of this trip—my nephew being twenty, that it was late summer and the weather was incredible, that I could get time off work to do it—all of these things would never happen in the same way ever again. I'm glad that I really savored them when I had the chance. And what can I blame this new awareness on? Yup. Surviving cancer.

Will I take Less Crap?

To paraphrase the great humanist and philosopher, Mr. T, I pity the fool who crosses you after you survive this. You will take a lot less crap after getting through cancer. There will, in all likelihood, be a much more piercing look in your eye than before. I found that after I had beaten this, things that were formerly very intimidating all of a sudden became much easier to deal with. After facing this kind of threat, the terrors of saying "no" to a salesman or speaking your mind clearly and concisely are much less scary. Once you begin asserting yourself in your relationships and making sure you get what you need, you'll start training people pretty darn quickly how to treat you. You may not have been able to stand up for yourself before, but (for those of us who were raised to turn the other cheek to the point of getting bloody) you are in for a bit of a treat. I found that I really enjoyed the process of redefining how people could or could not treat me and I hope similar positive things happen for you.

The Advantages of Being Yoghurt

Yoghurt has it easy. Stamped right on the bottom of its butt is its "best before" date. A tub of yoghurt knows that when

June 16 rolls around, it better have its affairs in order because if it's not eaten by then it's probably going to get trashed. It can judge its existence and live as fast or as slow as its "best before" date allows. If it has a lot of time it can afford to slow down a bit; it can say "Hey, I don't have to go to the big line dance in the vegetable section today, I can wait." Or it can know when it's time to get its will in order. We do not have that luxury.

Often we live as if our lives will go on forever. This might be a very nice illusion but in reality, our time is quite limited. We can get away with the self delusion of immortality because, unlike the fortunate container of yogurt, we don't know when we're going to kick off. Most people live out their days without really knowing how precious they are. Not you and I, my cancer-surviving friend. We know. We know that at some point everything that we have will be gone. I know this sounds horrible and you're thinking "Hey Rob, I thought you were going to uplift me here. I'm not sending you that box of dark chocolate after all." I firmly believe that knowing this is actually a great advantage. We now know that our time is limited and can live our lives with that wisdom guiding and enhancing our experience. What do I mean by enhancing our experience? How about making love more? Eating more chocolate? Drinking better red wine? Going out more? Getting more hugs? Giving more hugs? Going for more walks with your pet (even if it's a cat)? Making a telemarketer laugh? Essentially not waiting to live, but living *now*, for all it's worth.

Mediocrity? Bah!

You might find that you put up with mediocre experiences a lot less than you did before. If you're going to a restaurant and you really want the 12 oz steak medium rare instead of the diced hamster casserole, you're probably going to order the steak.

Steady as She Goes

It is essential to treat your precious relationships with care during this time. Make sure that even though you may be behaving differently and that you're reevaluating parts of your life, you remember that those close to you love you very much. Resist the urge to throw your whole damn life out. I can hear you already: "Wait a second Rob, a minute ago you were saying that we should go a bit nuts." Well, yes. In some areas you can allow for this, but in the realm of dear friends, family members and lovers, be careful. A damaged friendship or relationship can be difficult to mend.

Going through so much together, you might really see the people you love in a new light, feel remarkably close to them and be incredibly thankful to have all these great folks in your life. I certainly felt and feel that way. I know I've been funny* (I hope) and irreverent in this book but I've got to say that knowing I could count on my friends and family no matter what, helped me tremendously.

Some of the changes you experience will happen immediately and some of them may take a year or so to really settle in. Having more courage, being less fearful and appreciating each day will really make a difference in your life. I'm three years healthy now and I still find these positive changes rippling through my

world.

Who Knew We Were So Flexible?

"You have to leave the city of your comfort and go into

the wilderness of your intuition. What you'll discover
will be wonderful. What you'll discover is yourself."
—**Alan Alda**

Much as we like to think of ourselves as steadfast people
who are as unchanging as the statues on Easter Island, the
psyche actually doesn't work that way. We are much
more malleable and changeable than we would like to
think. Just as the sky is different each day, we can change
also. You might even notice shifts on a day to day basis
and think, "Hey, this is a bit different for me." Try not to
freak out; you might want to temporarily try a new
characteristic out. Let the changes happen and do your
best to forgive yourself along the way.

Watch for Fallout

There will be fallout with all of this. Growth does not
come without subsequent changes in your life and
sometimes the personal upheaval that goes with them.

Going through this, particularly with your partner, is
remarkably stressful. This doesn't mean you don't love
each other or aren't committed people. It does mean that
there is so much stress involved in an event like this that
sometimes a relationship can't take the strain. However,
with help, some couples find that they are closer than
ever and value each other even more than before. Sitting
down with a third party and having someone help you
navigate your feelings can make sure that you and your
loved one get through this with your relationship intact.

I found it really interesting that or a while after recovery I
really tried to "do the right thing" a lot. The only problem
was I didn't know what the right thing was anymore.
Since I felt so different, I didn't really have a moral
compass to guide me through decisions. My solution was

to just keep acting with integrity in the moment and to keep making decisions that were true for me at any given time; then I'd know I'm living with integrity and the rest of my life would hopefully fall into place. This was very much a "let the chips fall where they may mentality." I'd never done this before, and it caused a bunch of turmoil in my life for a while.

There is some confusion and emotional chaos as a result of being sick and I don't take that lightly, but once you live in a way that's true for yourself, a lot of the details end up taking care of themselves.

I've got to tell you that since my recovery I have had a series of adventures that I only dreamed of before I went through cancer. I've done some crazy things and have lived with a great deal more verve and energy than I did before. The biggest difference I think is that risk is no longer a four letter word. I'm not talking about going to Vegas and putting everything on red and hoping for the best (although hitting the high stakes Hold 'em room at the Bellagio would be a blast), I'm talking about understanding that risk and adventure are a part of life and knowing that the worst that can happen to you is probably not half as bad as what you have lived through already. Would I have had these adventures before I got sick? I'd sure like to think so but I must admit that after recovering my health, I jump at opportunities I used to only dream about because like our old friend yoghurt, I know that I have an expiration date.

"When the world says, 'Give up,' Hope whispers, 'Try it one more time.'"
—Author Unknown

Not all of the psychological changes you encounter will be positive. Being a ridiculous optimist by nature, I want to tell you about the good news as much as possible.

However, some of the long term effects of recovery took some adjustment. I went through a period of time when I was pretty scared of things. I'd wake up in the night thinking about how I'd been sick and wonder (quite illogically) if the doctors had missed anything. Then about a year after surgery, I would take a truckload of supplements, feel around where my thyroid used to be and just worry. This was all pretty natural. Now that more time has passed, a lot of these behaviours have faded and things are much easier. In some ways this fear was a bit of a counterbalance to the bravado that I had gained in other areas of my life.

For a while, I would just cry for no reason at all. I might be reading an email and would miss my friend who sent it and *Wham!*, I'd be bawling my eyes out. You might also find that you get really emotional at family gatherings; in the same way that older folks get very happy and teary when families are together, you might be emotional as well. Everybody else might be thinking "Hey why are they so upset? We're all just having dinner and eating dessert. Is it the lime Jell-o again?" The older people and cancer survivors are always blubbering because old folks and our club get it. We get that this thing called life is precious and we better enjoy it all now.

Like a Deodorant, You Will Be Soft and Strong

Ironically, when you get through this thing you will be both softer and stronger at the same time. How can that be? Well, you will probably be more sentimental and at the same time you will be tough as nails. This seems contradictory, but in actual fact it makes perfect sense. You see, you are more sentimental because you now probably value your family, friends and each hour of your life more than you did before. On the other side of the coin, things that would really piss other people off or leave them in a puddle of tears might now seem like no big deal to you. So in essence, you're kind of like a green beret who cries while watching long distance commercials. At least that's how you could describe yourself on an online dating site.

Chapter 12
Strategies for the Future

In this chapter:

Dark chocolate is your friend
Aunty Who?
Emphatically help your lymphatic system!
On the rebound
Ionic or ironic?

Things You Can Do Right Now

You can do a lot of things for yourself right now that will help you be healthier today and in the future. I know that when I was sick, I spent an awful lot of time feeling helpless and that there wasn't much that I could do for myself except wait around for treatment. It doesn't have to be this way for you. By making these very simple choices you will increase your level of health, the amount of energy you have and also reduce the risk of having cancer again. Most of this stuff is really easy to do and, as a bonus, is backed up by science.

Dark Chocolate is Your Friend

You heard me right the first time, but I'll say it again: Dark chocolate is your friend and so is red wine. Merry Christmas! I can hear you saying "What are you going on about Rob?" Well, let's talk about a little process known as Anti-Angiogenesis. This gets a little sciency (not a real word but it should be), so stick with me.

You see, when cancer is being formed in your body it needs an uninterrupted blood supply to sustain all that "out of control" growth. In order to get more blood to the malignant growth the body produces new capillaries. *Angiogenesis* is the process by which the body makes new capillaries in order to increase blood supply. In some instances this is useful and healthy for us. For example, in order to heal cuts and other wounds the body will increase its production of capillaries. However, when a person has cancer, the body uses angiogenesis to increase the blood supply to the malignant growth. This is not a positive process for the body to say the least.

Aunty Who?

Anti-angiogenesis is the process of impeding the growth of new capillaries. This is bad news for cancer, but good news for you and me. Interrupting, discouraging or impeding the supply of blood to a cancerous growth is nothing but beneficial and that is the process of anti-angiogenesis.

There are more than ten anti-angiogenesis drugs on the market at present. I'm sure that the drug companies have invested millions of dollars on research and development for these products but you don't have to give them any money or take any pills to reap the benefits of this process.

121

You can promote anti-angiogenesis in your own body just by eating certain foods that are available at any grocery store. In many cases, ingesting these foods can have as much positive benefit as taking the drugs without the expense or side effects.

Do you think I'm just making this up? Well, let's here it from Dr. William Li, the head of the Anti Angiogenesis Foundation. He is quoted as saying:

"We are rating foods based on their cancer-fighting qualities. What we eat is really our chemotherapy three times a day. We discovered that Mother Nature laced a large number of foods and herbs with anti-angiogenesis features."

Thanks to the awesome power of the internet, you can watch Dr. Li talk about his research in this very inspiring TED talk at this link; http://www.ted.com/talks/william_li.html

Some foods that have been shown to aid in anti-angiogenesis are:

Dark chocolate;
Red wine (1 glass a day for women, up to 2 glasses a day for men);
Blueberries;
Garlic;
Soy;
Green Tea;
Walnuts;
Salmon;
Lemons;
Tomatoes.

For a more complete list of foods that fight cancer you can go to http://www.eattodefeatcancer.org/

I don't know about you, but I am completely fine with

having all of these foods in my diet forever. This is considered to be some of the most profound research on cancer and diet in the last few decades and the best part about all of this is that everyone of us can help increase our level of health by making very simple choices at the grocery store and the dinner table.

Greens! Greens! Greens!

It turns out that your Mom and Aunt Suzie were right, eat leafy green vegetables! In a terrific book called "Fear Cancer No More" by Mauris L. Emeka, the author details a diet that can reduce your chances of getting cancer and increase your level of vitality. Mauris lost his wife to pancreatic cancer and did extensive research on diet and the best ways to support our bodies with nutrition. A diet rich in green leafy vegetables like raw spinach, collard greens, kale, Swiss chard and turnip greens is remarkably beneficial. Traditionally, we spend a lot of time stuffing ourselves with toxins like highly refined sugar, heavy starches and red meat. Hey, don't get me wrong, I love a good steak, but it's a really good idea to limit our intake of these foods. Emeka took four years to heavily research how the foods we eat can help prevent cancer and generally make us much more healthy. I recommend it highly.

Limit Sugar Intake

Eating a lot of refined sugar does some really lousy things to us, not limited to getting us fat. It also raises our PH level quite dramatically which in turn makes us much more prone to ill health.

Switch from Coffee to Green Tea

This was a tough one for me. I could go everyday
drinking five or six cups of java but it's actually quite
detrimental. Coffee raises our level of acid quite
dramatically. So a good alternative is green tea. Green tea
is amazingly good for us, has plenty of antioxidants and
as a bonus HAS SOME CAFFEINE IN IT! If you don't
want to completely give up coffee try replacing some of
your coffee intake with green tea in the afternoon and
you'll probably find that you really enjoy it.

Emphatically Help Your Lymphatic System!

Lymph, as you may or may not remember, is the fluid
that flows through our bodies and helps clean out our
systems. It does this by traveling around the body and
picking up waste and other nasty things in our systems so
they can be disposed of properly. Even though lymph is
remarkably powerful and important to our health, it does
not have a pump like the blood does, but relies on the
movement of our bodies to keep it circulating. Any
exercise that moves your whole body around will help
move your lymph as well. Walking, cycling, jogging and
swimming will all help your lymphatic system do its job;
however, one terrific way to move your lymph around is
to do a particularly beneficial thing called...

On the Rebound

Rebounding is essentially moving up and down on a
miniature trampoline. I'm not talking about leaping
through the air, doing somersaults and joining the circus
(although that sounds fun). Rebounding gets your body
moving, in a safe way that has many health benefits. It
increases your heart rate, is great cardiovascular exercise

and as a bonus, circulates your lymph.

This is a very effective way of helping your body detoxify as well as providing aerobic exercise that is easy on the joints. I use my rebounder everyday and feel much better for it.

In fact, NASA has gone on record as saying that rebounding is a more effective exercise than running. Here are some fancy quotes that back that up...

"Rebound Exercise is the most efficient, effective form of exercise yet devised by man." A. Carter summarized a NASA study in 1979, a study which NASA published in 1980 in the Journal of Applied Physiology.

NASA says, "...for similar levels of heart rate and oxygen consumption, the magnitude of the bio mechanical stimuli is greater with jumping on a trampoline than with running, a finding that might help identify acceleration parameters needed for the design of remedial procedures to avert deconditioning in persons exposed to weightlessness."

If it's good enough for NASA, it's good enough for me.

There are a couple terrific articles on rebounding here...

http://owen.curezone.com/healing/lymphrebounding.html
http://www.livestrong.com/article/282932-rebounder-lymphatic-exercises/

I have a Needak Rebounder which has proven very useful for the last couple of years. I use it to get my lymph moving gently in the morning as well as for more intense workouts. I love it. By the way, I do not have any business relationship with these folks other than liking their product. As always, be careful when starting a new exercise and check with your doctor to find out if it's right for you.

Hydrate!

Most of us actually drink much less water than our bodies need. The proper amount of water helps us detoxify and gets rid of a lot of the crap in our bodies. I find when I drink the right amount of water, everything works better. My digestion is easier, my skin feels better, I have more energy, and even minor aches and pains go away. Research shows we should drink an ounce of water for every pound of body weight. For a guy like me (I'm about 190. Really, humour me), I should drink about 190 ounces of water a day, which happens to be about three liters. Now that sounds like a lot. But if you drink a couple of glasses first thing in the morning and keep a bottle of water with you, then keeping properly hydrated gets a lot easier. At first, you'll probably go to the bathroom a lot, but after a while your body will get used to the idea that it's actually hydrated, so you won't have to pee nearly as much. In fact, when I'm drinking the right amount of water for my body, I'm actually very thirsty in the morning. I thought this was a bit strange until a friend explained it this way: many of us keep our bodies in a constant state of dehydration and so this feels normal for us and our body stops registering our feeling of thirst. However, once your body realizes it's not in a state of drought anymore, it lets you know how much it really needs by being thirsty. So, once you get rolling on having enough water, your body will let you know you're on the right track by asking for more.

Enough with the Cigarettes

Really? Are you still smoking? Haven't you heard and seen all the evidence on this? Put down the damn cigarettes. Oh I know it's highly addictive, but please stop. Every time you light up, the tobacco companies do a little dance and giggle like evil school girls because they know they are making money off of someone's horrible chemical dependence. Everything in your body is better when you stop assaulting it with nicotine, kerosene and a host of other chemicals too vile to mention. The good news is, the body can really clean itself out after you quit if it's given half the chance. In fact, your lungs will begin to clean themselves out almost immediately after you stop. Getting assistance to quit greatly increases your chances of success.

Ionic or Ironic?

I got introduced to ionic foot baths by my naturopath. An ionic foot bath uses a series of ionic pulses to stimulate your cells and help get toxins and other horrible things out of your body. Simply put, it works like this. You put your feet in a tub of warm water (very pleasant thank you very much) and then a wand is placed inside the water. This wand then draws waste out of your body through the pores in your feet. The pores in our feet are the largest in the body so it's much easier for waste particles in our system to pass through them. By placing our feet in warm water the pores in our feet open up and the wand can do its thing. While you sit there reading the paper, a whole host of things can be drawn from your system like excess lymph, cell debris, yeast, dead cells, and even some heavy metals and other toxins are drawn out through this fascinating process. At the end of twenty minutes or so, I am always amazed at the colour change in the water. After one of these sessions, I usually go home and sleep like the proverbial baby and when I wake up, I invariably feel great.

The machines themselves can be expensive but chiropractors and other health practitioners sometimes have them as an additional treatment to their main practice. I found the foot baths very useful to help get rid of the excess anesthetic and leftover toxins after surgery. Many people report benefits such as rashes disappearing, increased energy levels, increased sex drive, a lessening of chronic pain, better joint function and increased athletic performance. Once again, do your own research and find out if this is a good choice for you.

Chapter 13
But I Thought I Was Done!

"Life is a great big canvas, and you should throw all the paint on it you can."
—**Danny Kaye**

In this chapter:

A rugged hope
We are in this together
How would you treat a friend?
Signing off...

A Rugged Hope

To be honest, I already had the end of this book written months ago but upon reading it again I found that things had changed for me and I needed my last thoughts to be a little different. I think that's how this whole thing goes: we think we're done and we find we have a little further to go. We might get through the physical aspects of this disease and then we have to deal with how this thing affected our psyche or our relationships. During the healing process this drove me crazy. There was always another thing to deal with, another test to have done, another doctor to see, another "all of a sudden" to get past. This journey was longer than I thought and had implications way beyond the health of my physical body. In fact, I found the physical part to be straightforward and the effects on my life to be much trickier to deal with.

However, I have to tell you that there is hope here. Not the kind of syrupy, greeting card hope where there's a bunny with a caption that says "Everything will be just fine!" but the kind of hope that is a lot more down and dirty. A hope that understands there are days that are really difficult and times that are hard, but also this hope knows that on the other side of those difficult times there is a life for you, and that new life might even have some positive qualities that it didn't have before.

Life after dealing with this thing called cancer can be pretty good. Different certainly, but very good. In my own instance, life is richer now, relationships are deeper, I enjoy each day so much more. Would I gleefully volunteer to go through this thing that shook my life up on virtually every level? Absolutely not. But I will tell you that it is worth it to get through this. It is worth seeing it through the difficult nights and the fear and the pain to make it back to a healthy life again.

"Hope is patience with the lamp lit."
—**Tertullian**

We Are in This Together

There are many times when this process is lonely, when it seems like you just can't go on. Please know that when that happens, many of us who have been through this are with you in spirit. We know how courageous you are being everyday when the whole world thinks that you look "fine" but you're really just putting one foot in front of the other and hoping for the best.

Everyone's story is different with this disease. Yours will certainly be specific to who you are, just as mine was. I hope you find hope and encouragement along the way, that you have great medical care and get the support you need to help you on your journey. In a way, everyone who goes through this is family. We are joined by our common experiences and our struggle with this event in our lives. As I mentioned before, we are part of a club, we are veterans of a private war that we have fought. Only those of us who have been through it know what it is like and although our stories are different, we are joined by the common threads of strength, perseverance and courage that we know we need to be healthy again.

Along the way, please be patient with yourself, your body and those you love.

Get yourself as much support as you can. If you're sad, that's fine. If you're angry, that's alright too. If you need help, ask for it. Imagine if you had a friend going through this, wouldn't you give them all the love, support and second chances they needed to feel better? Of course you would, so please give that to yourself as well.

I started this book as a letter to a friend and I hope you know that I do consider you that. I know that we have probably never met, and possibly never will, but I offer what I have written humbly, not as an expert certainly, but as someone who would like to make this journey a bit easier for you.

I hope you continue to heal, and that you are able to encourage yourself during the tough bits and celebrate the progress that you will surely make when things get better.

I wish you all the best.

Love,
Rob

Chapter 14

For Caregivers: Before Treatment

** This portion of Kicking Cancer's Ass is intended for people helping family or friends going through cancer. Please feel free to hand this to them now, or heck, keep reading it yourself if you want. **

"Act as if what you do makes a difference. It does."
—William James

Hello Caregivers,

If you are accompanying a loved one who has cancer on a journey back to health, you are also in for a ride that has many twists and turns. The person you care about may be your lover, a family member or even a very close friend. In any case, I guarantee that you will know them and yourself in a different way after this experience. I also want to tell you that I have tremendous respect for you for going through this with someone you care about. You might be as angry, scared and befuddled as they are on occasion. I'm here to tell that's completely OK. We all know this is a serious subject. It's so serious in fact, that laughing at it occasionally can really help.

In this chapter:

Relax! You already know this
Listening, your best tool
How to prep for the hospital

Relax, You Already Know This.

I understand that helping someone you love through a health crisis can seem like a huge undertaking, but many of the skills and qualities you will use, you have used many times before. Chances are, you have helped someone you love who has been scared, tired or sick. I'm guessing you've held someone's hand and told them it's going to be OK. All of these things will be useful in the days ahead. You simply haven't yet called these things "looking after someone who has cancer."

Along the way, you will do some things that are very natural and normal for you; you will probably pick up some new skills as well. In either case, your "Loved One With Cancer" is very lucky to have you around.

Why Should You Listen to Me?

I have unique experience as both the caregiver and the person recovering from cancer. I had my cancerous thyroid removed on Feb 1 of 2006 and recovered over the next few months. My girlfriend at the time had the very same disease and surgical procedure on November 1st of the same year. I know, I was as surprised as you are. The first thing that came to my mind of course was that something very strange was going on. So I wondered if this had something to do with what we ate, where we slept, the clothes we wore, the cups we drank out of or even the massive electrical wires that went by my house

(They don't actually. But it would have been easier if they had, I could just look at them and say, Ha! I know why this happened. It's the damn hydro wires!).

So, when we went back to the same surgeon who had operated on me (a man named Dr. Freeman, whom I consider the Wayne Gretzky of thyroids), I looked right at him and asked what was up. He assured me that there was no connection between our cases and that if we had lived a thousand miles apart we would have come down with the same thing at the same time. I'm not sure if I believe this one hundred percent, but it did give me some degree of comfort. I was ready to move or burn all my clothing, or burn my clothing while moving, just to stop what was going on in our lives.

Thus began the second half of my journey with cancer where I became a caregiver. This of course, was very different from having the disease itself and had a whole different set of challenges that left me with some very valuable insights into caring for someone who is getting treatment for this disease. I'd like to share these with you now in the hope that it makes things easier for you and your loved one.

"I am always doing that which I cannot do, in order that I may learn how to do it."
—**Pablo Picasso**

Listen

You are going to do a lot of listening. This is probably the simplest and yet most helpful thing that you can do. You will get a lot of practice at this skill all the way from the earliest parts of this journey right through to the point where your loved one gets back to health. From the first time the person you're caring for gets the *possibility* of the big "C" dropped on them, they will have a lot to say. It will do them a world of good if they can express it to someone they trust and if that someone is you, then you will hear all about it. This isn't as hard as you think it's going to be. Just sit and be your empathetic self and listen. You might have to ask a question or two to get them going but once they do, they will just roll along by themselves. They may go from tears and despair one minute to somber acceptance the next and then back again in a heartbeat. The best thing you can do for them is stay present, respond and hold them if they need it.

To keep them going, you can use a bit of reflective listening. This is remarkably easy to do. You just take a bit of what they just said and reflect it back to them. They will, in all likelihood want to expand on what they said and before you know it, they'll be talking more than me after five cups of coffee.

First, Here's How Not to Do This...

It's about a week since the two of you have learned about the diagnosis and the initial shock has worn off. You're on the couch watching some stupid show on TV like "Washed-Up Celebrity Dance Marathon" when your loved one starts to talk about his/her condition. It might go something like this...

Them:
Oh man. This really freaks me out.

You:
Uh huh.

(You grab some more Fritos and wonder how long it took the wardrobe people to spray those costumes on.)

Them:
Uh, I'm kind of scared…I might have cancer.

You:
Yeah, you said that. I get it. Shhhhh. TV's on.

Them:
You bastard!

They run out of the room crying. You feel like crap, but hang on; you're a good person, so instead of doing that, let's try it again. You open up the conversation and give them your full attention by doing something a lot more like this…

You're in front of the TV again, this time watching that new game show "America's Biggest Root Vegetables."

Them:
Oh man. This really freaks me out.

You:
Hmm?

(You grab the remote, turn off the TV and turn to face them.)

Them:
I mean, I might have cancer. I'm really scared.

You:
Yeah, you're really scared…

Them:
Yeah! I mean what did I do to deserve this? This is awful! No one in my family has had this. What if they can't cure me? What am I supposed to do?

They begin to cry and you hold their hand or hug them. It's that simple. Your primary job is to be present and empathetic, and besides, you can always TIVO the root vegetable show for later on.

You Don't Have to Cheer Them Up!

Many people feel they have to cheer their loved one up in this situation. I certainly understand that impulse, but in this case there is so much stress and sadness in dealing with a diagnosis of the big "C" that they need to release these feelings in a healthy way. Talking to you about it and crying is a great way to do this. If it feels a bit uncomfortable, stay with it. They may have been very stoic at work and around other people, but at some point all that pressure needs to be released. Whether they are your sibling, parent, friend or partner, it is a real compliment to you that they trust you with their vulnerability. It's important to avoid the temptation to "shush" them, and instead to give them a safe space for those feelings to come out.

At every stage in his or her journey the person you're caring for will need to let off steam and it will be excellent if he or she can do it with your support and help. Now please note that I am not saying that you should take whatever they give you. If they become abusive towards you or direct their anger your way and you don't feel it's appropriate, call them on it. You are not a doormat and if you let yourself be one it will come back and bite you later on. What you can do is be very supportive and help them release this stress in a way that respects both of you.

Here is a Possible List of Things to Say
We will get through this.
I love you so much.
You're doing really well.
You have the courage to do this.
Whatever happens I will stand by you.
How are you feeling?
Whatever it takes we will find a way.

Can you tell me more about that?

So, you're feeling....? (fill in the blank with what they've just said)

...And Things Not to Say

You're blocking the TV.

Sorry, gotta go wash the car.

Wow, how did you manage to get cancer?

I told you to quit smoking/not eat meat/live next to power lines.

How does this affect me?

I know it sounds ridiculous to even have to mention this, but you'd be surprised how some folks handle this diagnosis. Listening in a nonjudgmental and supportive way can really help the whole situation.

Prep for the Hospital

If surgery or treatment is in the cards for the person you're helping, then there are some practical things that you can do to help get him or her get prepared.

Packing the bag for the hospital and making sure you have food and supplies ready for their return are two very practical ways to help them out. It will be a lot easier to take care of that now than it will be later, when they have returned.

Some people with cancer really want to look after everything and get incredibly organized before they go for treatment. Some, however, are too frightened to do anything and may need more of your help than usual to prepare for a trip to the hospital.

Ask them who they want to have visit while they are there. If there are people they really want to see, give these individuals a call beforehand and let them know that if they dropped by the hospital it would be really appreciated.

A couple of other questions might be whether they want you to spend the night at the hospital as well and what kind of food would they like to have at home after surgery. These simple forms of preparation will not only make things easier in the days ahead, it will also help them know that they are not alone in this experience, and that realization will help your loved one in every stage of healing. So: Listen. Offer support. Express a bit of love. It works magic.

Chapter 15

For Caregivers: At the Hospital

"A hero is no braver than an ordinary man, but he is braver five minutes longer."
—Ralph Waldo Emerson

In this chapter:

You're on deck!
Your skills will come in handy
Know your nurses!
Email to the rescue
Expect a shift
Getting out the door

You're on Deck!

When you get to the hospital, you will really shift gears. Very likely, this will be the time when the most demands will be placed on you and you will be the most active. Don't worry about being perfect; just deal with whatever is right in front of you the best you can. In fact, your just being there will be a huge help. No matter how tough or stoic your loved one appears to be, he or she will be VERY glad that you are present.

When they arrive at the hospital, they will check in with a nurse and then they'll probably be taken to a room where they'll be asked to change into a gown. That's really where the hospital experience starts for them. All of a sudden they are a patient in the eyes of the hospital and everyone else. This can feel dehumanizing and frightening, as all of it now becomes very "real."

Remember when I said that you'll need to draw on a lot of your strength at points during this ordeal? Well this is one of the times. You will have many roles while you are at the hospital, especially if the person you care about is going to be there for a while. You will be a diplomat, protector, counselor, keeper of the ice chips, medical interpreter and, at times, a jester.

If you're the closest person to the patient, the doctors and nurses will talk to you about all of the pertinent medical info. They may fall into medical jargon on occasion, and if they do, don't be afraid to say "Can you explain that a little further please?" or "What does that mean?" so you understand what's going on. It's very tempting to nod like you understand when they've explained things too quickly but it's completely OK to slow them down and ask for clarification.

When your loved one is prepped for surgery or treatment, try to stay with them as long as you can. When I went in for surgery, I had someone with me right up until I went into the operating room and it was a very big help. After they go into surgery, don't be surprised if you completely fall apart emotionally. You have been holding a ton in and have been strong for a very long time so you might cry your eyes out for a while.

And Now the Waiting Game

During surgery there won't be much for you to do. The hospital staff is taking care of everything so you can just relax for a bit. Find out when the earliest time is that they'll be out of surgery and after you do that its a really good idea to go down to the cafeteria for a while. Just have a coffee or tea and relax as much as you can. Even better, try to have a friend or family member with you at this point. This person will be your support system and comfort. It's a great time to go and spend some time with them and give yourself a break.

A bit before their surgery is scheduled to be completed, you'll probably be directed to the Surgical Waiting Room. You will be surrounded by other nervous people who are also waiting on their loved ones. Finally word will come down and you'll be told their condition, hopefully by the doctor himself. Remember to breathe deeply and write down notes if you need to, so you can recall the details later on.

While you are digesting the news and keeping yourself together, your loved one will probably go to the Surgical Recovery room for a while, where they will be watched very carefully to make sure that they are stable after the operation. If they were under a general anesthetic, they will most likely be unconscious or fading in and out. When they are well enough, the decision will be made to take them back to their room.

You'll have to wait while your loved one is wheeled there. Now you may or may not be able to see them after surgery as they may not be in good enough condition to even have a quick word with you. If it's any consolation, they will in all likelihood be quite medicated and thus not in pain, but also probably not very coherent. If you do get a bit of a visit, it will probably be short. Just give their hand a squeeze, tell them you love them and that they did very well.

Brace Yourself

When you see them after surgery, you may be in for a bit of a shock. They might look kind of rough depending on what kind of surgery they had and how they came through it. It's important to remember that what you do and say while they are semi-conscious or even completely unconscious is very important. They may be actually quite aware of what's going on around them, even if they look as though they are completely oblivious to their environment. I can still see my Dad in my hospital room really trying to hang on to his self-composure when he first saw me. That was OK. I just thought to myself "Man! This must be pretty bad if my Dad looks upset." Keep yourself as positive as possible during this time and offer some encouraging words like "You did it. You're done surgery. You did really well." And "Just rest now, everything is going to be alright." And if you really want to challenge yourself to keep from bawling, say "I love you so much and am very proud of you." If this is too much for you, just standing there and holding their hand speaks volumes.

After surgery they may be in rough shape and their whole body might hurt. How they lie on the bed, how the pillow fits under their head: all of these things might be a bit uncomfortable. So you might want to ask if they need anything shifted or adjusted. Even turning from one side to another can be a welcome relief if their own body weight has been pressing down for quite a while.

Ice Chips

Ice chips can be remarkably comforting as well. If they are receiving drugs intravenously and getting most of their fluids through a tube in their arm, chances are their mouth will be remarkably dry, so a trip down to the ice machine might be just what the doctor ordered. After clearing it with the nurse, get yourself a cup full of ice chips and put a few in their mouth, making sure, of course, that they are not at risk of choking. They might want some ice chips a few times an hour because this is one of those small things that can make a big difference in their level of comfort.

If you stay the night or into the wee hours of the morning, you will be on a bit of a vigil. The hospital will become much quieter, the guests will be gone and there will be fewer nurses and staff around. Many of the patients will just be sleeping comfortably. If they are having a good night's sleep and are quite unconscious, my advice is to go home and get some much needed rest. If you can, stay around until your loved one is sleeping. Just very gently say goodnight to them, let them know you're going to go for the night and then wait for them to settle in before you slip out the door. Getting ready to leave the bedside of a loved one who has just had surgery is some very tough stuff. Take heart. These are the hard parts that you've heard about and you can get through them. Just put one foot in front of the other and you will get through it. Remember that they are getting good care and that you need to be healthy and rested for the next day.

Smaller Chunks!

One very useful thing that helps me when things are tough is to break time down into smaller chunks. What do I mean by that? When things seem overwhelming and I might not be able to handle looking at the coming week or even the next day, I break time into smaller, more manageable bits. Instead of thinking of the whole day, I might think about only the next hour that I have to deal with. For instance, I might think "All I have to do is drive to the hospital." or "All I have to do is make sure that they are as comfortable as possible right now." The old adage of taking a day at a time can be reduced to an hour-by-hour way of looking at things. You can even think of time in ten minute increments. I mean, you can handle the next ten minutes right? You might want to keep doing this until things get easier, and before you know it you'll be back to thinking about next week again.

And Now, an Inappropriate Comedy Break

Here are a few fun things to do while you're in their room and they're sleeping comfortably.

1: Switch the charts of other patients and watch the fun as people get the wrong drugs.

2: Find a doctor's gown and go diagnose the loud guy in the cafeteria.

3: Give yourself a sponge bath.

4: Find the intercom and say with great authority "There's a code Magenta in my pants!"

5: Try to sell the nurses your products from the new and improved Amway!

6: Cram as much Jell-o into your mouth as possible and make your own "Jackson Pollock" on the wall.

7: You and a buddy grab a couple of wheel chairs and do a drag race all the way down to obstetrics.

8: Grab the chief of Thoracic Surgery and give him noogies until he yells "Uncle."

If you do decide to stay the night, make yourself as comfortable as possible, have a novel or trashy magazine ready and feel free to eat some of the candy that came via the day's visitors. Then settle in. The chairs aren't bad, and if you're really lucky, the next bed will be empty and you can sleep on top of it and get an hour or two of rest yourself. If you are really fortunate, they will have a cot for folks like you who want to stay overnight.

Know Your Nurses!

I know that nurses are incredibly professional and empathetic, but people are people and if you can address them by their first name and know a couple of things about them, it can really help. So be friendly and as calm as you can. In fact, I have it on very good authority that to get "in" with the nurses all it takes is a coffee run. If you're on a vigil, or it's late in the evening, drop by the nurses' station and ask if anyone wants anything. A quick trip to the Tim Horton's (or Starbucks, if you prefer) where you get the nursing staff a double-double and a chocolate glazed will do wonders for your reception while you're there. Of course make with the "thank you"s and small talk as well. It's very basic stuff to remember but it will build a positive relationship with the professionals who are helping the one you love.

Listening: The Sequel

The person you are caring for will have stories to tell after they get out of surgery. It might not happen at first, but in a day or two they will want to tell you how it was for them. They will tell you whether or not they were scared, if it hurt, what the first night was like, how the drugs are, and, if they have the strength, a myriad of other things. Hold their hand and listen. Offer a comment or two to keep them going. It's very important that they express themselves, as they have just gone through a heck of a trauma. Chances are they will tire themselves out really quickly when they talk, so when they seem to flag, encourage them to get some rest and assure them that they can tell you all about that later. Looking back on this stuff, it sounds kind of easy and basic but this may be some of the most centering, nurturing and generous time you two will spend. Ever.

Sometimes your loved one will tell you things they won't tell the nurses because they don't want to be a bother. You might find out that they are in some pain. If they are, you can tell the nurses for them. Say something like "Buella's in some pain right now, is there anything we can do about that?" Be as non-confrontational about it as possible. It's tempting to snap and say something like "Why haven't you given them enough morphine, dammit?" But be cool: you're in a relationship with these folks and it helps everybody if it's a good one.

The Balancing Act

The key to getting through this part of the process (and the whole thing, for that matter) is balancing the needs of the person you're caring for with your own needs. You'll be giving a lot to them for a long period of time, so when you get the chance to do something for yourself, do it, whether it's a walk, a movie, a really good cup of coffee or phoning a friend. You're not made of stone and you have needs yourself, even though you may have been ignoring them for a while. This isn't being self-centered at all. This is making sure that you are staying healthy yourself emotionally and physically. You could look at it this way: you'll be able to help them a lot more if you're in good shape, so treat yourself well.

Visitors

There will likely be people who really want to come and visit at the hospital. One of your duties will be to arrange for visitors to go in and out of the room, all the while making sure that your loved one isn't too tired to see people. As the point person, you may need to manage how these visits go and how long folks stay. This can take a fair amount of juggling. If you have a lot of visitors coming and going through the room make sure that it's not too much for your loved one. If you have ten people visiting, it may be a bit overwhelming. Periodically ask them if it's OK or if they want to sleep now.

Again, it can be a tricky balance. Having friends and family there is a real boost for them psychologically. Knowing you're loved and having folks around is great, but there will be a time when it's too much. Just let everybody know that the person you are caring for is happy that they came around and that now it's really time for him or her to rest because it's been such a big day. You might say, "You know, it's great you came, thanks a ton for your support, but she's really tired now. Can I pass on a message?"

Visiting Hours Are Over

The patient might not even be aware of it themselves, but they might be completely worn out from visitors and be barely able to keep their eyes open. That's when it's time for you to step in and let everyone know it's time to go. The guests can all come back another time or, if they are disappointed, let them know that they can really help out by swinging by the house in a week or two and visiting then. Their company (or cooking skills or laundry ability) will come in very handy at a later stage of recovery.

It will be obvious if your loved one needs to rest. Their speech will slow down or their energy level will drop. When that happens, suggest to everyone in the room that it's time to wrap it up.

"A good heart is better than all the heads in the world."
—**Edward Bulwer-Lytton**

Email to the Rescue

An easy way to deal with communication before and after treatment is through an email update. You can tell the story of the surgery in one message that is sent to family and friends, which will save you answering the same questions again and again and let people know as much or as little as you like. The ones I sent were on the longish side, and I wrote two or three over the course of my loved one's surgery and recovery.

Here's an example of what you might want to send out after surgery...

Hello Everyone,

First of all, thanks so much for all of your help and good wishes in the last while. As you may or may not know, Buella has been going through a tough time and had cancer surgery yesterday. She is currently resting well and we are all a bit tired out after dealing with the hospital. She was remarkably strong (if not a bit nervous) when she went into the hospital on Tuesday morning, but after getting settled in, things seemed a bit better. We had to wait a couple of hours because things were a tad slow that day. Once she got into surgery things went smoothly. The doctor says she is resting comfortably and anticipates that Buella will be able to go home on Sunday morning. We are keeping visitors to a minimum right now so that Buella can get her strength back. If you would like to visit or chat when she is more able, that would be great. Thanks so much for all your thoughts and prayers. Hope all of you are well. Gerald.

This will really help you out. It will answer a bunch of questions for people, will help build a support network for you later on, and will also let people know what is up with their very good friend Buella. Let this serve you as much as possible. Tell people what you want them to know. My updates were pretty detailed as I really wanted loved ones to be part of the process and to have people be involved as time went on. Email updates can also be a way for you yourself to hang onto the reality of the situation while it's going on. Later, you might want to read them over again and they will help you remember in more detail what happened. You'll be able to look back at it and say "Hey that was really a hard time. Man, things are so much better now." This kind of measuring stick of progress can be a really big help.

You might want to send out another one of these after your loved one gets to a different stage of recovery: "Buella is now eating solid food and is very happy to be back home and sleeping in her own bed. She loves the cards and DVD's all of you sent. Many thanks."

I Can Feel the Earth Move!

Every relationship has some sort of aspect of power to it, whether it's between siblings, lovers or a parent and child. I believe in the altruism of love as much as the next guy but whenever two people get together there is eventually some kind of agreement about who has more influence in the relationship. This manifests itself in small instances such as whether you go to the movies and see *The Screaming Fists of Death* or *The Whimsical Diary of Never Ending Love Poems*. On a grander scale it affects where you live, who you hang out with, and whether you buy good chocolate or the cheap stuff.

So, I would assume that the two of you have worked that out to some degree. You may be the one in the driver's seat, both literally and figuratively, or your partner may be the one primarily in control. Heck, you might even have it worked out so that you take turns doing this, in which case I say "Bravo!" When you get on the merry go round known as "caring for someone you love who has cancer" things are going to change. You will have much more influence and control than you did before. Up until surgery or treatment, you will be dealing with and supporting someone who is very definitely in emotional and physical turmoil and quite frightened.

When they go to surgery or into treatment there will be another shift in the relationship as well. From the second you walk into the hospital, you might become the point man or point woman for the whole thing. Going in for surgery or an invasive treatment is essentially a profound loss of control for your loved one, so a lot of that power is shifted to you. Everything from where to park the car, to getting info from the doctors and nurses, to deciding what to tell family and friends may rest on your shoulders. I'm not going to lie to you, this is not easy. However you will be able to handle it. Seeing someone you love in a state of distress will call up some very deep and profound resources within you that you may not know were there and, as in any crises, we often find unseen strength at our disposal. In all likelihood, you'll have the opportunity to use these resources as your loved one goes through treatment.

A Natural Shift

And again, when you bring them home, you may be doing a lot for them, from keeping track of the meds to preparing the food to helping them to the bathroom. I myself can't say that this was a walk in the park, but I do know that it was the perfect thing for me to do at the time. The person you love may have very little in the way of resources right after treatment, especially if he or she was under general anesthesia, so you will be doing most of the decision making and offering a great deal of support to ensure that they can heal properly.

After your loved one begins to recover, this balance may shift again. Chances are there will be a new depth and understanding between the two of you. The stuff that pissed you off before may seem remarkably trivial. Those fights over the laundry and who is going to feed the zebras will fade in their importance as you watch your partner get back to health again.

Crisis Mode

During and after surgery, you will be in crisis mode. You will be battening down the hatches and navigating through the storm. There may not be time for you to feel anything while this profusion of events occurs, but at some point you will probably have a natural burst of emotion. This could manifest itself as anything from a bit of crying to misdirected anger to a deluge of sobs.

While I was looking after someone with cancer, I got through the first and second day at the hospital no problem. I dealt with everything that presented itself and was hopeful and positive through the second day she was there. All of this changed when I showed up at the hospital the morning she was to be discharged and saw that she wasn't feeling well at all. All the progress of the day before seemed to be gone and she looked like (and was) someone who had gone through major surgery.

Seeing someone I loved very much in that condition hurt and quite frankly scared the heck out of me. A friend of ours gave me a hug outside the hospital room and I broke into these huge sobs. I cried like a baby. I needed to. It was probably the best thing for me at the time, as I had gone through the last few days with a stiff upper lip while saying "Damn the torpedoes." Your proverbial dam may burst as well. You will be asking a lot of yourself in the days to come and you will need to let off some steam as you go along.

Leaving the Hospital

In addition to being a place where people have medical procedures and eat bland Jell-o, a hospital is also a large bureaucracy that needs to be negotiated like a trip down a set of rapids. The best thing you can do is keep your eyes open and be prepared to change direction at any time. At some point, a doctor will make an examination and say that your family member or partner can be checked out and go home. Leaving the hospital is actually a project in itself. You may need some help on this day. In fact, I'll go out on a limb and say you will *definitely* need some help on this day. Get a very good friend or family member who you can rely on and ask them to come along for the ride (for me it was my buddy Gord). A doctor will give an exam and give the nurse the OK. Then there may be some confusion about when you actually will leave, so if this happens, go to the nurse and get the scoop.

When the person I was caring for left, it was quite confusing. A nurse came in and said "She can't go today, she's not well enough." A few minutes later a doctor came in and added "I don't think she'll be going today." Then her actual doctor looked at the chart and said, "OK, she's ready to go." With every one of these pronouncements, we would be excited or saddened, but when we finally got the word from her actual doctor we figured she was well enough to head home.

You're probably going to be helping them into their clothes (your loved one, not the doctor) to get them ready to go. Everything they do will take more time than you think. Just buckle up and get ready to exercise a lot of your patience and a double helping of your strength. An orderly may come by and offer a wheelchair for you to use during checkout. Take him up on this offer. Even if the patient is strong and feels fine, their level of stamina will probably be quite low. If they balk, say something like "I know you don't need it but just do it as a favor for me," and that will hopefully do the trick.

You Will Need a Buddy!

The person you're caring for will have to sign some papers, get some medications from the pharmacy, and then you'll be on your way. This is where your buddy comes in. Your loved one will very obviously not be at full strength, so if you have a car there (be prepared to curse the exorbitant hospital parking rates) you will need your buddy to get the vehicle while you stay with your partner in the lobby. When you all get in the car, in the hospital loading zone, it's good to have another person around to keep the vehicle running while you help your loved one to get in. A hospital loading zone can be a very busy place and you will be very happy to have them there to help you out. So drive carefully and slowly and remember that your goal is to get your loved one home with as little pain and discomfort as possible.

Chapter 16
For Caregivers: At Home

In this chapter:

There's a reason why it's called "Home Sweet Home"
Dealing with the phone
You've done this before
Managing meds
Better than Christmas morning
Care for the caregiver
You're my hero!

There's a Reason Why It's Called "Home Sweet Home"

The first thing that will probably happen when you get your partner home is that he or she will make it to bed and fall immediately asleep for a long period of time. They will be so happy to be in familiar surroundings and will be so tired after the ordeal of getting checked out of the hospital that they will just fall unconscious.

You might be a bit nervous about looking after them and think "Oh man, I'll have so much to do!" When they fall asleep, sit down and rest a bit, maybe get your favorite food ordered in, and congratulate yourself on a job well done.

If you are lucky enough to have a job where you can get a bit of time off work, then that will be remarkably useful right about now. Take some vacation days if you can, or have no shame at all in telling your boss "I need some time off to take care of my wife/husband/boyfriend/ sibling who is recovering from cancer." William Randolph Hearst himself would find it hard to turn you down on that one. They will probably ask if there are things they can do to help. Tell them "Sure! How about an office fundraiser for a weekend away when this is all over?" Really. Ask.

That White Cap Looks Good on You!

Once you get them home and they are safely in bed, you will probably realize that you are now a nurse. Oh, you might not be registered but you will definitely be holding down the job. You might be a lumberjack, a systems analyst or even a systems analyst who specializes in lumberjacking, but for the next while, you will be wearing a metaphoric white cap. You will learn how to do this very quickly and I'm guessing you'll do it well. You'll be able to pull this off with the help of our old friends, empathy and strength.

The Phone

While you are lying slumped on your couch with a hot cup of tea or a stiff drink and listening for any sound from the bedroom where your loved one is recovering, people will probably call with good wishes for a speedy recovery. In fact, there might be such a flurry of calls that you want to turn the ringer off for a couple of days. You can put an outgoing message with some info on it that explains the situation. Something as simple as "Hi, It's me. I just wanted to let you know that surgery went well and Buella is recovering well at home (and working on that name change). I'll be returning calls in a couple of days but for now we're pretty busy. If you'd like to leave a "Get Well Soon" message please do so at the sound of the beep. Thanks!" Beep. This should take care of a lot of the explaining for the first while and you can then return calls at your leisure.

Relax: You've Done This Before

Depending on what shape your partner is in, you may have to do a lot for them. This can mean everything from giving them meds at the scheduled times, to prepping meals, to feeding them, to helping them in the bathroom, to changing dressings, changing them, and of course, skimming the tops off the chocolate pudding. This might seem daunting at first but you've actually done a lot of this before. If you've ever looked after someone who has had a nasty cold or a case of the flu, then consider that your training. It's quite similar in a lot of ways. You just have to be available, open and generous to the situation. You will probably fall into a routine after a while.

Keeping Track of Medications

I suggest making a chart with the medications on it so you can keep track of what has to be taken when and then check it off when it's been done. This will help a lot, as it's very easy to forget if things were taken an hour ago or three hours ago. As long as it is clear, concise and you can follow it, then it's a good chart. Keeping track of meds can be a bit tricky at times, so a simple tool like this can go a long way:

Better than Christmas Morning

Here's a something I'm pretty proud of that will help a ton. It's like Christmas morning for someone who is recovering from surgery or treatment. When you get home and you're taking care of your family member, partner, or friend you might want to send out an email to a huge list of folks they know.

This could go something like this...

Dear Everybody,

As you may or may not know, Buella is healing from surgery. She had a tough time of it in the hospital and is now recovering at home. The very scary bit is now over and we are in the longer slower period of getting back to full health. Many of you asked if there was anything you could do; well now there is! It would be very helpful and generous if you could drop a get-well card in the mail for Buella. She would love it. It doesn't even have to be a get-well card; it could be anything that you think she would like. This will let her know that she is not alone right now and will really brighten her day. The address is...

Extra credit for anything homemade!

Many thanks,
Gerald

Send this out to virtually everybody on Buella's email list and your list as well. You will be amazed at the response. Folks you haven't heard from in years will send something in the mail that day. In a few days, cards will start rolling in and your Buella (who will hopefully be up and around and with a different name at this point) will be endlessly entertained and touched by an outpouring of love. I am not exaggerating. This can be such a lonely time that knowing people are thinking of you and loving you is more beneficial than any drug. These cards will be read more than once and can (and should) be pulled out on days when things are a bit tough. Again, it's important to remember that this is not an imposition on people at all. They will really want to help and will compete to be the funniest, warmest and most significant. As a bonus, you will be given incredibly high praise. You will hear "Oh my god, she is so lucky to have you helping her" more than once.

Generosity

If ever you wondered when in your life you would have a chance to be generous then this is it. You will give a lot and (because I'm assuming you're a good person and probably generous by nature, otherwise you wouldn't be reading this right now) you might wear yourself out a bit by looking after your loved one. Your own needs have probably been on the back burner for a while now. Let's face it, for the time before treatment you have been the rock, the shoulder to cry on, the person listening when you just couldn't listen anymore. You've also been the one who, when friends see you, has to hear "How's Buella doing?" over and over again.

Bring on the Double Chocolate Explosion!

Since they've been home, you've helped them go to the bathroom, cook meals, done the laundry, written emails, probably fielded phone calls, even talked to crazy Uncle Jack whom you can't stand. You think Superman is tough? Ha. Let's see him deal with this. That's why I

159

recommend that as soon as your loved one is able to be on their own for a few hours (which is probably sooner than you think) you need to go out and do something really decadent for yourself. My favorite thing to do at a time like this is getting a massage. Go for an hour and get somebody to really rub the kinks out of your body. You will feel tremendous. If you're worried about the money, justify it by saying "Hey, I'm just making sure their caregiver is in top form."

Care for the Caregiver (That's You!)

Here's a brief list of things you could do for yourself.

1: Go for a massage

2: Have lunch at your favorite restaurant

3: Take a buddy to a movie

4: Jump on your bicycle for a quick spin

5: Go swimming

6: Go to your favourite ice cream store and order two scoops of your favourite ("burnt marshmallow" and "double chocolate explosion" come to mind)

Essentially find something that you love that has nothing to do with cancer recovery and do it. You'll feel a lot better and you'll be able to look after them again sooner than you think.

These Boots Were Made for Walking

It's also a great idea to take the person you're caring for on a lot of slow walks. Easy exercise is great for them right now as it helps the body re-acclimate itself to activity again. It also assists in getting rid of any anesthesia that may be floating around in their body by speeding up the circulatory system. Walking is a simple yet profound activity that can have some tremendous benefits. So, go on a nice slow stroll everyday with them if you can.

Sex

"Don't knock masturbation - it's sex with someone I love."
—Woody Allen

OK, we're going to talk about sexuality right now. If you are in a romantic relationship with the person you're caring for, then during the last while you have probably been experiencing a profound lack of sexual attention. There will be a lot of energy going from you towards them but it is very doubtful that it will be of an erotic nature. You will spend a lot of time nurturing them but there won't be much coming back to you in other ways (and by other ways, I mean hot, steamy sex). I don't really know what to say here other than that you may be "looking after yourself for a while" and that is about the size of it. It can be a frustrating thing for folks but it is part of the deal when you are looking after someone who has gone through a surgery or another significant treatment. Their body is probably just not up to it at all and they will most likely come around again, but for now, you will have to wait.

You're My Hero

Even though I don't know you, I have a ton of admiration for you. To look after someone going through this takes a great deal of courage, empathy, patience and, of course, a truckload of love. Now, you might think to yourself

"There is no way I can do all of this" or "How can I look after someone else when I am so scared that I'm going to lose them?" Those feelings are completely natural in your situation but I'm here to tell you that you can get through this. This is a marathon and not a sprint, and as each day brings new experiences and new challenges, you will meet them and deal with them one step at a time.

There are times in this journey when you will be pissed off and tired of looking after somebody all the time. You'll just want to go to a movie or out to dinner but you might not be able to. To top this off, the person you're looking after might be completely ornery and seem a bit ungrateful. If this happens, get a friend to spell you while you do something purely for yourself. You've been a superstar for a long time now and you just might need a break from the whole thing.

On the opposite side of the coin, there will be times when you will feel like you can deal with whatever happens and the level of intimacy and love you feel for the person you're caring for will be overwhelming. Sometimes, both of these extremes can happen in the same five minutes. Take deep breaths and remember that better days are coming.

This journey is an adventure of the highest order. I'm not talking about an adventure on the high seas with pirates and treasure, but an adventure of the spirit that can take a lot of patience, love and strength. You have my profound respect for going through this with someone you love. Those of us who have experienced it know what it takes.

God bless you for it.

Rob

About the Author

Robert Hawke is an actor and writer. He co-wrote and performs the internationally renowned play NormVsCancer: A Terminally Funny One Man Show, which received a Canadian Comedy Award nomination for Best One-Person Show.

Rob is associated with The Centre For Innovation In Complex Care at the University Health Network and is co-lead of the Patient Empowerment Program. Rob has performed NormVsCancer for physicians, nurses, medical students, cancer patients, their families and the general public. If you would like to see NormVsCancer performed, please contact Rob.

Rob shared in a Gemini Nomination for his work on CBC TV's SketchCom. He is an alumnus of The Second City comedy troupe. He lives happily in Toronto with his wonderful wife and ridiculously small dog.

Connect with me online:

Twitter: RobertHawke

Facebook: Robert Hawke

Web: www.normvscancer.com

email: robhawke@gmail.com

8842661R0

Made in the USA
Charleston, SC
19 July 2011